The

Beginners

The Ultimate Beginners Guide to
Decrease Blood Pressure Naturally,
Improve Your Health,
Lose Weight, and Burn Fat
In the
Most Simple, Healthy, and Scientific way

Kathleen Moore

Table Of Contents

Introduction

Congratulations on taking the first step towards better health!

In recent years, we've become all too dependent on the pharmaceutical industry for our health. We've come to believe that we can pop a pill to solve any health problem and have failed to take responsibility for our own decisions. And, many common health problems including serious diseases like diabetes, heart disease, and cancer, have been thought to be "normal", due to aging.

What if the real story was completely different and you actually had control over many of your long term health outcomes? Yes, aging and death will get us all in the end – but you can choose to be healthy and age well or you can sacrifice your health to diseases believed to be "inevitable" and become a prisoner to drugs and endless doctor visits.

The medical establishment is slowing becoming aware that what we put into our mouths every day might actually determine how well our body functions! Yes, it's a shock to many, but your diet and nutrition have a huge influence on so many things. On top of this, we now know that nutrition can influence whether or not you develop dementia or Alzheimer's disease, and how well you can get around and take care of yourself when you're elderly.

It's true that some things are genetic and your family history might loom large. But even then, taking control of your diet and nutrition will go a long way toward promoting your overall health. You are not a victim and the fact that you've chosen to read this book indicates you're ready to take charge of your health!

So why is the DASH diet important and something you should consider trying? The answer is simple. DASH was originally developed specifically to deal with high blood pressure which is sometimes called *hypertension*, but it turns out that multiple health issues like being overweight, developing diabetes and many of the other issues that we've mentioned are all related. At their root, they at least in part meet at a common cause. So while DASH had a specific intent – to lower blood pressure – it also improves health across the board, promoting weight loss, improving blood sugar, and reducing cholesterol. Here is an added bonus – in recent years evidence has been mounting linking high blood sugars to cancer (lots of insulin in your bloodstream contributes as well). Since DASH helps you lose weight it *may* even lessen chances of cancer.

Enough of the pep talk. It's time to get started. Let's find out what the DASH diet is all about, how and why it was developed, and how you can use it to improve your health!

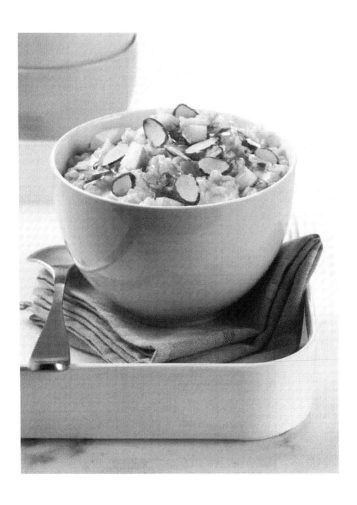

Chapter 1: What is the DASH Diet?

In this chapter, we will explore the history of the DASH diet. First, we'll learn why the DASH diet was developed and the theory behind it. Then we'll take a look at how early trials of the DASH diet developed and what the results were. We'll talk about the general benefits of the DASH diet, which we will explore in more detail in later chapters.

What Does DASH Mean?

DASH simply means for **D**ietary **A**pproaches to **S**top **H**ypertension. Hypertension or having a high BP, is a common but very serious health problem that was once called the "silent killer". By doing damage to blood vessels and key body organs, it can lead to ill health and even death. Some of the victims of high blood pressure have been world famous – U.S. President Franklin Delano Roosevelt was among them, sadly living in a time just before the first pharmaceutical treatments for and understanding of hypertension came about. He died in 1945 near the end of the Second World War, and some of the first effective treatments for high blood pressure were developed just a few years later, in the 1950s.

High Blood Pressure: The Silent Killer

Roosevelt died from a cerebral hemorrhage, which basically means a blood vessel in your brain bursts and it fills with blood, killing off your brain cells. He had multiple health problems – and most of them could be traded to his high blood pressure. We measure blood pressure in mm of mercury, which is abbreviated mm Hg. The reason this is done is that historically (and often still today) scientists measure pressure by seeing how far a thin column of mercury will rise inside a narrow glass tube, or capillary. Mercury is metal but its liquid at room temperature. The properties of mercury made it ideal for measuring pressure.

Blood pressure has 2 parts, the systolic and diastolic. Systolic blood pressure is the number at the top and diastolic blood pressure is the lower or the one at the bottom. So your blood pressure is given like this:

Blood pressure = systolic/diastolic

Systolic and diastolic blood pressures are measured in units of mm Hg, and not to get into a mathematics lesson, but we need to know this to understand what we're reading - the units cancel since we have a ratio. So you can simply refer to the ratio when describing overall blood pressure while understanding that individually each number is measured in mm Hg.

Systolic blood pressure measures the pressure in your blood vessels when the heart is contracted. In other words, it's the pressure when the pump is forcing blood through the arteries. That's why it's a larger number.

Diastolic blood pressure measures the blood vessels when the heart is at rest. While it's a smaller number, a high pressure when the heart isn't pumping can indicate serious health problems!

FDR's blood pressure was routinely above 200/100, and may have been as high as 300/195! Have you checked your blood pressure lately? It's probably not nearly that high.

If your blood pressure reached 200/100 or 300/195, it would be considered an emergency. Back in those days, FDR was allowed to continue his usual routine in daily life. Today, 200/100 would be considered an emergency requiring a visit to the emergency room while 300/195 would be considered absolutely catastrophic. And of course, it was – when his blood pressure got that high he ended up dying.

Let's briefly talk about pipes and pumps so that we have some understanding of how blood pressure works. You can imagine a water pumping system with a pump that pushes the water through the pipes. Different pipes will lead to different conditions. Without getting into the physics and engineering behind it, you can understand that pressure will go up if the pipes are narrow, compared to pipes with a wider or larger diameter. Also, to get the same amount of water through, the pump has to work harder or expend more energy to get that water through narrow pipes than it does through larger pipes. The water also travels at a higher velocity and what happens if you break open the pipes? The more narrow the pipes the more forceful the water gushing out would be.

Your circulatory system – and we are focusing on arteries and veins in this case – is pretty analogous to this. Actually, its more than an analogy, your heart is a pump and your arteries are pipes. However, there is a key difference when comparing this to your basic water pumping system described above. Your arteries have some flexibility that metal or PVC pipes found in your plumbing don't have. They can contract and expand, based on many factors. Some of these factors are related to the immediate environment. Remember how narrow pipes help push fluid faster and more forcefully. What happens when you're exercising? Your body tissues and muscle need more oxygen –and hence more blood. So your arteries are going to contract to help get that blood where it needs to go as quickly as possible so you can run or whatever effectively. In other words when you exercise your blood pressure goes up.

Conversely, if you're totally relaxed or meditating your blood pressure goes down.

Many things can lead your blood pressure to go up or down, not just exercise or relaxation. Some people are simply pre-disposed toward high blood pressure because of their genetics, or as we say in common language their family history. As you age, your bodily functions are not as efficient as they were when you were young, and this impacts your circulatory system as well, so the blood vessels may not relax as well as they used to and your blood pressure may creep up as you get older.

But there are many environmental factors that influence blood pressure. In particular, drugs or substances that are stimulants tend to raise blood pressure. A stimulant can be thought of as something that puts your body in a fight or flight state, and so it tightens up your blood vessels. Some over the counter drugs like Sudafed which work in part by tightening the blood vessels in your sinus and nasal passages can cause higher blood pressure in certain sensitive people. Illegal drugs like cocaine and meth can raise blood pressure to dangerous levels and as a result, cause massive damage to the circulatory system if used regularly over extended periods. The New York Times reports that many people who indulged in cocaine use during the 1980s are now showing up with major cardiovascular problems, including a high risk for a brain hemorrhage and also bursting of a major artery in your gut area, which is known as an abdominal aneurysm (before it bursts).

On the legal front, the use of tobacco products is also associated with high blood pressure and the resulting damage to the cardiovascular system that tightening of those pipes we call the arteries can lead to. This is largely due to the presence of nicotine, which like cocaine and meth is a stimulant (though it's of a milder variety).

Cigarette smoking, in particular, is tightly linked to a higher risk of high blood pressure, abdominal aneurysm, and cerebral hemorrhage. If you're a smoker, one of the best things you can do for your health is to quit now – and the elevated risk of lung cancer isn't the only reason for doing so.

Even drinking caffeine, in the form of coffee, tea, or energy drinks, can impact the blood pressures of some people. Some folks are more susceptible than others, and it also depends on how much you drink and how rapidly. For most people, coffee and tea will have no impact, or only temporarily raise their blood pressure mildly. But others will be more susceptible. Some energy drinks, which might have more concentrated levels of caffeine, may be more of a problem. There have been reports of some people even having bleeding in the brain and nearly dying after consuming large amounts of energy drinks.

Hypertension – How Does Diet Come Into Play?

Of course, drugs and stimulants are not the only environmental factors that impact blood pressure. Fluid retention can also be important. When a patient is suffering from fluid retention, this means that blood moves through the arteries at a slower pace. Remember we noted when you exercise blood moves through your arteries at a faster clip – helping to give your tissues, cells, and muscles the extra oxygen and fuel they need to function at a higher level. So you won't be surprised to learn that if you're suffering from fluid retention and blood flow is reduced, your tissues, cells, and muscles aren't going to be getting the oxygen and nutrients they need to function properly. But your body doesn't take this sitting down – it tries to adjust. Specifically, your kidneys can recognize reduced blood flow and respond in turn. The kidneys will cause the release of certain hormones that lead your body to retain sodium and fluid (so it's like a feedback cycle – retain fluid, kidneys then cause your body to retain more). One thing that happens when you've got fluid retention is the fluid in your blood increases in volume – so you're trying to pump more fluid through the same pipes. What does that do? It increases blood pressure.

Electrolytes

We don't want to make your eyes glaze over by going too deeply into the science, but a few basic facts will help you understand high BP and the DASH diet. First, we need to know what an *electrolyte* is simply put, it's a substance in your body that is "ionized". In other words, it carries an electrical charge. Electrolytes are very important when it comes to the basic functionality of the body's systems. In particular, they are involved in nerve function or neurotransmission and they help regulate how the blood vessels behave.

The main electrolytes related to nerve function and the function of your blood vessels are:

- Sodium
- Potassium
- Calcium
- Magnesium

We don't need to know the details, but we can understand how these work in the body in the following way:

- Sodium tightens your blood vessels, or put another way tends to increase blood pressure. Sodium is also closely associated with fluid retention.
- Potassium, calcium, and magnesium are associated with relaxing the blood vessels or put another way they tend to lower blood pressure.

- Calcium also contributes to lowering of blood pressure.
- Sodium, potassium, magnesium, and calcium are all important for the proper function of the heart muscle. For example, a magnesium or potassium deficiency can lead to palpitations or problems with heart rhythms. Severe deficiencies of any of these minerals can even lead to heart arrhythmias that are so drastic they can be fatal.

It's important to understand that sodium (or salt, which is how we get sodium through our diets) is not an evil or bad thing. You must have salt in your diet – without sodium, your body would not function properly. In fact, recently a woman in Israel suffered major brain damage following a fruit juice only diet. Doctors explained that it was the lack of salt which caused her health crisis. Fruit has lots of potassium and magnesium but very little sodium. For more info on the story see "Fruit juice diet sends a woman to the hospital with brain damage".

The article about the fruit juice diet makes something clear – the *balance* between sodium, potassium, calcium, and magnesium is what's important.

Stroke

We've mentioned that FDR died of a brain hemorrhage. Basically, one or more blood vessels inside his head had become weakened over time from his high blood pressure. When they become weak, their structural integrity becomes compromise and they can break – just like a water pipe being forced to carry more than it's designed to handle.

Brain hemorrhage or bleeding in the brain is one kind of stroke. You can also suffer a stroke caused by a blood clot. Another side effect of high blood pressure is that your blood vessels become more calcified and stiffened over time. This leads to clots and blockages leading to heart attack and stroke. Moreover, your blood vessels are less able to respond to stress since they lose some of their pliability and plasticity. So if you get angry, causing a surge in blood pressure, if your system can't handle the increased load and you could end up having a stroke or heart attack. This can also happen when engaging in vigorous physical activity.

Direct links between blood pressure and mineral content of the diet

One of the first indications that diet could have a big impact on blood pressure came from observations of people in Japan. As you know, the Japanese diet, while very healthy overall consisting of lean meat, copious amounts of vegetables, and rice, also uses a lot of salt. Soy sauce which is very high in sodium is practically used with every meal, and sauces like teriyaki are also very high in sodium.

It's not surprising that the rates of stroke are a bit higher in countries like Japan where more sodium is consumed. However, that isn't the entire story, and what scientists found out would be a clue leading them to discover how diet could be used to help control blood pressure.

It turns out that in some regions of Japan it's not just sodium that's consumed in copious amounts, but they also eat apples. And what do apples contain? A lot of potassium and magnesium. And guess what – the rates of stroke in these regions were far lower when compared against Japan as a whole.

Enter the DASH Diet

Many years later, when scientists had continued to gain knowledge of the influence of the electrolytes sodium, potassium, magnesium, and calcium on blood pressure, scientists in the United States began working on developing a diet that would address the imbalance of these minerals found in the standard American diet. In the early 1990s, this research came to heat at the National Heart, Lung, and Blood Institute or NHLBI, which belongs to the National Institutes of Health or NIH, part of the federal government in the United States.

The impetus for the diet came from a simple fact about the way people in the United States were eating. While we weren't piling on the soy sauce, like people in Japan Americans were consuming far too much sodium on a daily basis. And more to the point, they were doing it out of balance with potassium, magnesium, and calcium. Many Americans are deficient in all three, but magnesium deficiency is particularly common.

With this in mind, a diet was developed not to eliminate sodium from the diet, but to consume it in appropriate amounts and in balance with adequate levels of potassium, magnesium, and calcium. A key fact when it comes to this issue is that the average American consumes 3,400 mg of sodium per day. The nutritionally adequate level of sodium intake is believed to be closer to 2,300 mg per day.

The impact of sodium intake on your health depends on many factors. Some people are more sensitive to it than others, and other dietary components can mitigate high sodium intake. That said, the researchers set out to design an ideal diet that balanced all the important electrolytes you need in your body. In order to get adequate levels of potassium, magnesium, and calcium, they determined that the diet should include large amounts of fruits, vegetables, and dairy.

While the diet was not designed for weight loss, we'll see later that the diet does lead to weight loss and control of weight for many people.

The diet was tested in large studies conducted by NIH. A good study doesn't take place in isolation, so the researchers actually divided study participants into three groups, each group getting its own diet to follow. Then at the completion of the study, they could be measured and compared to see if the DASH diet had any impact.

At the time of the original study, the low-fat mantra was in vogue. Since that time we've found that there are good fats and bad fats, and focusing solely on fat consumption often misses the point. For example, it's been found that while researchers thought higher amounts of saturated fat intake are bad for heart health, the reality is that's only true if you're also consuming large amounts of simple carbohydrates. The truth is not as simple as it was believed to be in the 1960s-1990s when it comes to nutrition.

That said, a low-fat approach does improve health when it's done properly and in balance with other important dietary components – something that is done to high precision on the DASH diet. One of the key advantages of DASH is it's simplicity.

Returning to the study, the first group of the study was placed on what is now known as the DASH diet. The diet sought to increase:

- Consumption of lean protein.
- Potassium, magnesium, and calcium.
- Dietary fiber.

By increasing the amount of lean protein consumed, this helps reduce saturated fat intake while making meals more substantial and satisfying. As we've seen, potassium, magnesium, and calcium contribute directly to reducing blood pressure and maintaining a healthy cardiovascular system, provided that sodium isn't reduced to unhealthy levels. Finally, dietary fiber helps with the absorption of carbohydrates, reducing blood sugar spikes. It may also help remove excess cholesterol from the body and helps maintain digestive regularity.

Magnesium and potassium are also found alongside calcium in dairy products. Hence, the diet was also designed to incorporate regular consumption of low-fat dairy products in addition to large amounts of fruit and vegetables. For bread, pasta, and other grains, study participants consumed "whole grain" varieties. We'll explain what "whole grain" really means in a later chapter.

An important component of the DASH diet was to limit sodium intake. The key word here is limit. As we noted above, sodium is necessary for the proper functioning of the human body, but we simply eat too much of it and not enough of the other minerals in our diets. There is already a lot of sodium in most natural foods, and so the simple act of salting food can lead to excess sodium intake. Processed foods like crackers and deli meats contain large amounts of sodium. The researchers allowed study participants to consume limited amounts of sodium and they were given salt packets to use which had carefully regulated amounts contained within.

Careful consideration was given to meat intake. While the DASH diet allows the consumption of red meat, this is only allowed on an "occasional" basis (including pork). Poultry and fish consumption are the preferred protein sources for DASH. Of course, the diet is readily adapted to a vegan or vegetarian lifestyle, beans and legumes can be substituted for meats without significantly changing the diet.

Sweets are allowed but in moderation. We will explore the specific amounts allowed from all the major food groups in a future chapter.

The DASH diet study actually had two "control" groups. A control group is used to compare some item you're studying against a group that doesn't have the item to see how much impact it has and whether it's really significant. The first group followed the standard American diet for the most part but had significantly increased consumption of fruits and vegetables with no other changes. This was important because it would allow researchers to determine if the DASH diet in its entirety was necessary to maximize benefits or whether fruits and vegetable consumption alone could regulate blood pressure.

Finally, a "full-on" control group would consume the standard American diet without any interventions.

When the first study was completed, researchers found out that both the DASH diet and the one which simply increased consumption of fruits and vegetables lowered blood pressure. However, the impact of the DASH diet was far more substantial. In particular, while the diet worked for all study participants it had the most impact on people who have hypertension.

The DASH diet was able to lower systolic blood pressure by an average of 11.4 mm Hg. It was also found to lower diastolic blood pressure by an average of 5.5 mm Hg, not as dramatic but still significant. These numbers were comparable to those obtained using medications in some cases.

Now, remember that the second diet increased consumption of fruits and vegetables, but otherwise people continued to eat whatever they were eating prior to the study. While this was not as dramatic as the results seen with DASH, it was beneficial. On average study participants in the fruits and vegetable group saw their systolic blood pressure drop by 2.8 mm Hg and their diastolic blood pressure by 1.1 mm Hg.

Of course, those following the standard American diet with no intervention experienced no beneficial changes.

This study demonstrated that the DASH diet can work as well as medications in some people, and works better than consuming a lot of fruits and vegetables with no other changes.

What About Weight Loss and Diabetes?

As we'll see, the DASH diet strictly limits servings and portions but does it in a very easy to follow way. By regulating overall food intake and specific numbers of servings for each food group, the diet naturally leads to weight loss for those who need it. As a side benefit, the focus on whole grains and lean proteins helps those who are pre-diabetic or even those who have full-blown diabetes. These issues will be explored in more detail in later chapters.

What is a good blood pressure reading?

Many folks know that having high blood pressure is bad for their health, but they aren't so clear on the details. So let's lay them out here.

For the most part, doctors consider healthy blood pressure to be around 120/80 or lower. Obviously, it can't be drastically lower than this, very low blood pressure can cause lots of problems on its own such as making you pass out. However, some doctors are taking a harder line, suggesting that your blood pressure should be 115/75 to be considered "normal". It's not entirely clear that having it that low, however, is consequential for health.

When your blood pressure inches upward into higher ranges, you're considered to have so-called "pre-hypertension". This is a range at which there aren't going to be any short term health consequences (and maybe none ever) but that you're in danger of running into future trouble. It's also considered a range where you're more likely to get things under control by making lifestyle changes rather than having to go on medication. For systolic blood pressure, the pre-hypertension range is generally considered to be 120-129 mm Hg. For diastolic blood pressure, the range is 80-89 mm Hg.

For all blood pressures higher than these values, medical professionals divide them into three ranges. These are:

- Stage 1: This is between 140/90 and 150/99. Whether or not you will be placed on medication or not may vary by doctor, but most will probably put you on a mild or low dose blood pressure medication.

- Stage 2: This is considered far more serious with implications for overall health. The range here is 160/100 and higher.
- Emergency: If your blood pressure tops 180/110 then this is considered a medical emergency and a trip to a hospital is warranted.

Doctors may also consider the range between diastolic and systolic blood pressure. The difference between the two is called the pulse pressure. So if you have a blood pressure of 135/90, your pulse pressure is 135 mm Hg – 90 mm Hg = 45 mm Hg. Since 120/80 is still considered the ideal blood pressure, you can see that a pulse pressure of about 40 mm Hg is what would be considered healthy.

A high or low pulse pressure can indicate problems, especially for patients over the age of 60. If the pulse pressure is high this indicates a high risk of future heart attack or stroke. This holds more strongly for men but is true generally. If pulse pressure is greater than 60 mm Hg, the patient is considered to be at higher risk of a future heart attack. However, a high pulse pressure may also indicate other health problems related to the cardiovascular system like leaky heart valves.

Low pulse pressure can indicate health problems as well. That can indicate that the heart is not working properly, has become weakened.

While a pulse pressure of 40 mm Hg is a good value when we are talking about blood pressures in the normal range, it can't be taken in isolation. If you had blood pressure of 170/130, your pulse pressure would also be 40 mm Hg, but a patient with blood pressure of 170/130 is at a lot higher risk than one with blood pressure of 130/90, or even someone with larger pulse pressure but lower overall values, like 140/90 which would be a pulse pressure of 50 mm Hg.

High pulse pressure can be caused by damage to the aorta, which is the main artery supplying the heart. If you have heart disease which means plaque buildup from fatty calcium deposits in your arteries, they stiffen. Stiffened arteries don't respond to changes in the force of pumping blood as well as normal arteries, leading to the higher pulse pressure.

Blood pressure medications not only reduce overall blood pressure but may also help lower pulse pressure.

A Brief Overview of Blood Pressure Medications

Let's briefly review some of the major classes of blood pressure medications prescribed by doctors and how they work.

Diuretics

These are the oldest of blood pressure medications. Basically, they cause your body to eliminate fluid and sodium from the body, by excess urination. By reducing fluid and sodium in the body, they reduce the amount of fluid in the blood and hence reduce blood pressure. While they work, they aren't as effective as newer medications and also have some problems associated with them. For example, it's not just sodium that gets taken out of the body – all that fluid will take potassium with it too.

Beta Blockers

Remember that pressure isn't just due to the size

of the pipe, the action of the pump and how forcefully it pushes fluid through the pipes can impact pressure as well. Beta Blockers work on this by acting directly on the heart, to reduce heart rate and the force with which the heart pumps.

Ace Inhibitors

ACE is angiotensin-converting enzymes. Basically, they make angiotensin, a hormone that makes blood vessels contract, or become narrow, raising blood pressure. By blocking the production of the hormone, it reduces blood pressure. It's not blocked completely, only reduced.

Angiotensin II Receptor Blockers

These drugs work on the blood vessel narrowing hormone as the ACE inhibitors but in a different way. They block some angiotensin molecules from binding to the blood vessels, to reduce the narrowing effect.

Calcium Channel Blockers

While calcium is beneficial for many aspects of health, it increases the force of contraction of the heart, and for people for which this is a problem contributes to high blood pressure. Calcium channel blockers reduce this effect.

Alpha Blockers

In short, alpha blockers help the blood vessels dilate, or relax. This reduces blood pressure.

Vasodilators

These also work to help the blood vessels dilate, but by a different mechanism than alpha blockers.

Adrenergic Inhibitors

These drugs are older and work by blocking mechanisms in the brain that tell the blood vessels to constrict. They are only used rarely these days if other medications don't work because they have a lot of side effects.

DASH Diet leads to healthier kidneys

The health of your kidneys is closely tied to high blood pressure. It's also tied with diabetes. Later we'll see that the high blood sugars associated with diabetes can damage organs like your kidneys. This, in turn, can actually lead to high blood pressure. In turn, high blood pressure can also damage your kidneys. The DASH diet addresses both of these problems. The blood pressure problem is addressed directly by the diet. By helping you maintain normal blood pressure levels, the DASH diet helps keep your kidneys healthy. When it comes to diabetes, the DASH diet, which is based on whole grains and high fiber foods, can help control, eliminate, or prevent diabetes. As a result, patients who follow the DASH diet will have healthier kidneys as a result of their blood sugar being under control.

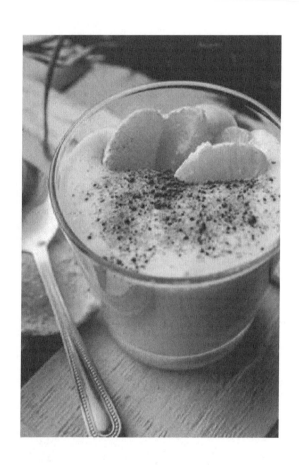

Chapter 2: The DASH Diet Food Pyramid

Now that we know a little bit about where the DASH diet came from, let's take some time to get an overview of what is actually in the diet and what the basic rules are that you should follow. To do this, we'll utilize the DASH diet pyramid.

Let's get started by looking at the pyramid and exploring how it's different from the USDA's recommended food pyramid:

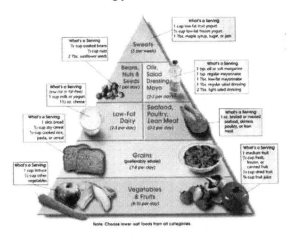

The first thing that should catch your eye is that the DASH diet is one that emphasizes fruits and vegetables. These should be eaten in large amounts and constitute the bulk of your food consumption.

Next up we have grains. Whole grain foods are required for the DASH diet, so no white bread, white rice, processed white flour, or regular white pasta. You can find high fiber and high protein versions of white pasta, that may be acceptable, but you shouldn't consume it unless it's specifically noted as such. Whole wheat pasta and pasta made from so-called ancient grains like einkorn or quinoa are perfectly acceptable.

You also eat grains in copious amounts, however, they should be consumed at a slightly lower level than fruits and vegetables.

The next step up the pyramid is not only smaller but it's a shared level, indicating that these are foods that should be consumed in more moderate quantities. Starting on the left, we see dairy products. The original DASH diet recommends that you consume low-fat dairy, however, in recent years, there have been studies done with dairy products that were full-fat varieties like whole milk. Surprisingly, the research has shown that DASH dieters may fare better when consuming whole-fat dairy products. Those that do so show superior blood lipid results as compared to regular DASH dieters.

Dairy products include milk, cheese, and yogurt. Typically you're not going to be consuming butter or cream, or even half-and-half while following a DASH diet.

Moving to the right, we see the meat category. On the DASH diet, at this level when we say meat we are only including poultry, fish, and other seafood. Red meat is allowed on DASH, however, it's an item to only be consumed in strict moderation. Poultry is eaten with skin removed. Due to their omega-3 content, you should be consuming fish at least a couple of times per week. Remember that the DASH diet was developed before there was much knowledge of omega-3 and the role of fish and omega-3 oils in reducing heart disease. If you are going to eat red meat – which includes beef and pork – it should only be eaten on a "now and then" basis. Think once a month, and the fat should be trimmed after choosing leancr cuts.

Next up, on the left, we have beans, nuts, seeds, and legumes. Despite your perception of these as being healthy foods, they are consumed on an even more moderate basis than poultry and fish. Nuts can include any variety, such as walnuts, almonds, macadamia, and cashews. The seed category includes items like sunflower seeds and pumpkin seeds, both of which are an excellent addition to the diet.

Legumes refer to peanuts, lentils, soybeans, and peas.

To the right, we find condiments and oils. On the DASH diet, these are more restricted than some people would like. Items that are allowed include margarine (not butter), olive oil, mayo, and salad dressings. Low-fat varieties are preferred but the regular editions can be consumed but in lower amounts.

Now we arrive at the top of the pyramid. This is where we find sweets. You can have small amounts of sweets, but when they say sweets they don't mean chocolate bars. Sweets do include small servings of sugar, honey, and syrup, as well as fruit-based yogurts. Frozen yogurt is also allowed as an occasional treat. At the time the diet was originally developed there wasn't nearly as much low fat and fat-free ice cream on the market, but those would have to be consumed in rare and very small amounts due to the added sugars.

It might surprise you, but the USDA food pyramid is actually a little bit different. Rather than having fruits and vegetables at the bottom of the pyramid, the USDA recommends grains as the food item to be eaten the most. This includes bread, cereal, rice, and pasta.

The next level or step of the USDA pyramid is occupied by fruits and vegetables. Above this, we find dairy and meats, with the "meat" category also including eggs, beans, and nuts.

At the top of the USDA pyramid, we have sweets and oils, to be consumed sparingly.

So the layout the differences:

- DASH recommends consuming most of your food in the form of fruits and veggies. The USDA recommends consuming most of your food like bread, rice, cereal, and pasta.

- While the amount of grains recommended by both isn't dramatically different, the DASH diet recommends consuming up to twice as many servings of fruits and vegetables as the USDA recommends.

- The DASH diet specifies low-fat dairy. The USDA makes no recommendations for this category. Also note what we said above, that some studies have found consuming full-fat dairy produces better results for DASH dieters.

- The DASH diet limits the consumption of beans, nuts, seeds, and legumes. The USDA recommends consuming in moderation but doesn't list them out as a separate category, classifying them with meat instead.

- The DASH diet recommends poultry, lean cuts of meat, and seafood. The USDA diet only recommends that protein sources be consumed in moderation.

- The DASH diet doesn't specifically mention eggs, while the USDA pyramid allows them without specifying how many to eat. Keep in mind that the original DASH diet was created during the "eggs are bad" era. Our recommendation is to treat one or two eggs as a serving of meat, and egg whites are more in line with the theme of the diet than a whole egg.

Whether or not you're following the USDA guidelines for diet – we suspect that the vast majority of people are not – the similarities between the DASH diet and the USDA diet recommendations are strong enough that most people find adopting the DASH diet relatively straightforward.

Low Sodium

The first thing to keep in mind is that the DASH diet is based on one central proposition – consuming a low sodium diet. Actually, that's not entirely fair because what is "low sodium" is actually based on our distorted pallet, which has been a condition by what is actually a *high* sodium diet. The DASH diet does not prohibit sodium at all – you're encouraged to eat enough salt to get 2,300 mg of sodium per day. Do note, however, that there is a lower sodium version of the diet which limits intake to 1,600 mg per day. This diet is an option for people who have more serious blood pressure issues, however, everyone should probably try the 2,300 mg per day limit first to see how it works for them.

One way to lower your sodium intake is to stop salting foods. Americans tend to reflexively reach for the salt shaker when their plate is set on the table. Why not try tasting the food first?

Especially when eating out, your food is going to be pre-loaded with salt. So the idea that it needs more salt is on shaky ground, to begin with, and you might find that it tastes just fine without adding extra.

Another option is to season your food with alternatives. These days the sky is the limit when it comes to seasoning your food, and from the exotic to the mundane, you can make your food a lot more flavorful without relying so much on added salt. Try spicy cayenne pepper, salt-free garlic powder, curry powder, or any one of what seems like a virtually endless array of options.

One interesting alternative is potassium chloride. Known as the table salt-substitute, potassium chloride gives you a similar type of seasoning that is 100% sodium free. It does have a biting taste to it but after you use it for a while you'll find yourself getting used to it and even enjoying it. Not only is this a no sodium alternative for seasoning your food – it's a great way to increase your potassium intake, which will help you reduce your blood pressure.

Some companies make lite salt varieties which are still sodium based salts but contain half the sodium of regular salt. These are made by combining potassium chloride with regular salt.

Recommended Servings

The DASH diet has the following recommended servings for each food group. You should try to follow them as closely as possible, but remember these are guidelines and as long as you're following the general principles of the diet there is no reason to beat yourself up over not getting everything exactly right.

- Vegetables: Have 4-5 servings per day (four is the minimum). One serving consists of a ½ cup of vegetables or a cup of lettuce. The truth is you don't need to worry about going over any limits with vegetables if we are talking about leafy greens (spinach, kale, arugula), or other green vegetables (broccoli, asparagus). However be sure to watch it with starchy vegetables like turnips, potatoes, carrots, and sweet potatoes.

- Fruits: You can eat 4-5 fruits per day (like vegetables of at least four servings). For whole, fresh fruits, one medium-sized fruit constitutes one serving. Frozen, canned, and dried fruits tend to have more concentrated sugar, so one serving is limited to a half a cup. Fruit juice, while providing many of the important nutrients found in fruit, also has concentrated calories and sugar, so one serving is limited to ¾ cup.

- Next, we have grains. While fruits and vegetables should be eaten in quantities of 8-10 servings per day, grains are consumed in slightly fewer amounts, recommended at 7-8 servings per day. When it comes to bread, one slice is one serving. Dry cereal, rice, and pasta come in at ½ cup per serving. Remember that the DASH diet recommends that you consume whole grains. So no white bread or white rice.

- Dairy: Now we consider dairy, which includes yogurt, milk, and cheese. The DASH diet doesn't allow you to eat butter, cream, buttermilk, or sour cream. You can have 2-3 servings per day. When it comes to milk and yogurt, a serving is one cup. A 1 ½ oz portion of cheese counts as one serving.

- Meat: To be consumed 0-2 times per day. A serving of meat is considered to be a 3-oz portion. This seems like an overly strict rule, a serving of meat is going to vary for say a 120-pound woman and a 200-pound man. In any case, use your own judgment, if you are working out on a regular basis you'll probably want more protein than they recommend. Any type of fish or seafood is acceptable on the DASH diet. Poultry is also acceptable provided that it's skinless. You can also eat beef and pork, there are no explicit instructions to avoid it. However, it's recommended that you consume leaner cuts of beef and pork. A good cut of beef that could be consumed on the DASH diet would be sirloin. You'll probably want to trim the fat when eating meat on the DASH diet, and red meat and pork would be consumed less frequently than poultry and seafood.

- Beans, Nuts, and Seeds: The DASH diet only allows one serving per day. However, beans legumes (peanuts, lentils, soybeans, peas) are excellent low-fat sources of protein. They also provide a lot of dietary fiber. Therefore you may consider eating more servings by substituting them for the up to 2 servings of meat per day. This also works well for vegans and vegetarians. Nuts contain large amounts of fiber along with copious amounts of potassium, magnesium, and some calcium and other minerals. Therefore it's safe to assume that eating a handful of nuts per day can be a good idea. The DASH diet defines a serving of nuts to be 1/3 of a cup. For seeds, which are also rich in important nutrients, the DASH diet recommends 2 tbsp per serving. A serving of beans (or lentils etc.) is a ½ cup.

- Oils, Salad Dressing, Mayo: You're allowed 2-3 servings per day. Light or low-fat varieties have larger amounts per serving. For salad dressing, 1 tbsp of regular salad dressing is a serving, but you're allowed 2 tbsp per serving for low fat or fat-free varieties. For low-fat mayo, you can have one tbsp. Regular mayo is limited to a tsp per serving. One serving of oil or margarine (butter is not allowed) is one tsp. The type of oil is not considered on the DASH diet, but note that it was developed long before the benefits of olive oil and avocado oil were known, so use your own judgment when deciding what type of oil to use.

- Sweets: Finally we arrive at sweets. You can have up to 5 servings per week, but the definition of sweets is a little bit restrictive. Maple syrup, sugar, or jam can be consumed at 1 tbsp per serving. One cup of low-fat yogurt with fruit is one serving of a "sweet", although until now you may have thought of yogurt with fruit as dairy, and not a "sweet". Finally, you can have a ½ cup of frozen yogurt, and it must be low-fat.

How Does the DASH Diet Compare to Other Diets

These days there are so many diets making the rounds it's going to be impossible to make a comparison between the DASH diet and all the others. But let's take a look at some of the most popular diets.

Atkins

The Atkins diet is a low carb diet, so it's very different from the DASH diet. Atkins advises followers to limit consumption of carbohydrates to 20 grams per day for the first few weeks, which is the "induction phase". This phase is designed to put your body in "ketosis" where you're burning fat rather than blood sugar for fuel. Over time, the restriction on carb consumption is relaxed, but following the Atkins diet, you will never consume the level of carbohydrates you will on the DASH diet. The

Atkins diet also puts no restrictions on sodium intake at all.

The Keto Diet

The keto diet is a version of the Atkins diet, or we should probably say that the other way around. The keto diet was developed many decades before the Atkins diet. Originally it was developed to treat children with epilepsy. Like Atkins, it's designed to operate on the principle of "ketosis", so you burn fat rather than blood sugar for energy. It also proposes a similar radical restriction of carbohydrate consumption, but unlike Atkins does so for the long haul. If you follow the keto diet you'd basically limit your carbohydrate intake to 20 grams per day or less for life. Unlike Atkins, keto also restricts protein intake, to about 15-30% of total calories. The keto diet makes no restriction on the amount of salt consumed, in fact, some keto experts advise consuming more salt.

Paleo

The "paleo" diet or as it's sometimes called the "primal" diet is based on the belief that primitive humans consumed certain foods (during the Paleolithic era) and that our bodies are designed to eat these foods. Whether their compiled list of foods is accurate or not is up for interpretation, but basically, you can think of paleo as Atkins with some add-ons that will up your carbohydrate intake but without consuming any processed or modern varieties. To see how this works, sweet potato is acceptable on paleo, but bread and pasta are not since they are foods invented by civilized man. While you can consume more carbs (or limit them, your taste) there are no specific rules for consuming fat and protein, and adherents often like to consume more fatty goods for the energy. They also strongly advise eating grass fed beef as opposed to standard beef which is fed grains. Like the other diets, salt is not restricted.

South Beach Diet

The South Beach Diet was very popular in the late 1990s but appears to have lost steam, being wiped out by Paleo and keto in the diet wars. To be painfully honest, the South Beach diet was a rip off of the Atkins diet and not really much more than a marketing ploy. It can be thought of like a modernized version of Atkins in the sense that at the time the South Beach diet was invented leaner meats were favored as that was in the middle of the fat is bad era. So the South Beach diet promoted low carb eating, but with lean cuts of meat.

The Mediterranean Diet

Like the DASH diet, the Mediterranean diet has gained a widespread following among medical and health professionals. However, as we reviewed earlier, the DASH diet was literally created by doctors who were doing research trying to treat blood pressure using diet. The Mediterranean diet, in contrast, was never invented by anyone. It's simply the way that people in the Mediterranean basin eat, and have been eating for countless centuries. It's not all that different from the DASH diet, except that it does not restrict salt, and encourages the consumption of some red wine. The Mediterranean diet also emphasizes the consumption of fatty type fish, such as mackerel and sardines, which are found in copious quantities in the Mediterranean sea. It also encourages liberal use of olive oil, and consumption of nuts, which is, in contrast, the restrictions on oil use in the DASH diet. However, the similarities between the two diets are strong enough that some nutritionists have been pushing a combination of the diet called the "DASH Mediterranean solution".

Readers may be interested in looking into the DASH Mediterranean solution, so let's take some time to review the food pyramid for the Mediterranean diet. Again, keep in mind that the food pyramid really isn't anything official, because this is nothing more than the native diet consumed in Greece, Israel, coastal Italy, southern France, Morocco, and of course Spain and Portugal, which are probably the two best representatives of the Mediterranean diet.

That said, based on the eating patterns of people in these regions the nutrition community has concocted a food pyramid. At its base are whole grains, including bread, rice, and pasta among others. Unlike the DASH diet, the Mediterranean diet doesn't offer specific guidance on serving sizes or number of servings per day, only relative servings between different food groups. Beans and nuts are actually often included with whole grains at the bottom of the pyramid.

Next, you're advised to eat large amounts of fruits and vegetables. On the next level of the pyramid, however, we find olive oil. This is a major distinction between the DASH diet –

which severely limits oil intake, even of healthy oils – and the Mediterranean diet. On the Mediterranean diet, you're advised to consume olive oil in large amounts. You can also consume related oils (those based on monounsaturated fat) like avocado oil.

The only recommendations for the lower 3 levels of the Mediterranean diet pyramid are that you consume them "daily", and that you have mostly whole grains, then fruits and vegetables in slightly lower amounts, and olive oil in slightly lower amounts.

Above this, we have fish and seafood. According to those advising this diet, you should consume them "a few times a week", but we imagine if you lived on the southern coast of Spain or Italy you might be eating more seafood than that. In addition to eating fatty varieties of mackerel, sardines, and anchovies, you can eat lean seafood like octopus, squid, and scallops.

Next, we arrive at eggs, cheese, poultry, and yogurt. The only advice given here is to consume them "daily to the weekly". For cheese and yogurt, there is not any specification of whether to consumer low-fat or regular varieties. We suspect that in traditional cultures regular, whole-fat varieties were consumed. There are no specifications to eat skinless poultry.

Finally, at the top of the pyramid, we have meats and sweets. By meats, in this case, they mean red meat and pork, and probably lamb which is very popular throughout the region. There are no restrictions on fat in the meat, however, you should be consuming "meats" in small amounts or monthly. Whether anyone living in the area actually follows the rules this closely is up for debate, of course.

So now that you know what the Mediterranean diet is, how would you go about combining it with the DASH diet? The first step would be to start with the Mediterranean diet and simply limit sodium intake to 2,300 mg per day. Second, you can follow the portion guidelines advised in the DASH diet, along with with the servings per day guidelines.

You may stop there and achieve great results for your health. If you're not getting results, you can cut back on olive oil (which may be healthy, but being fat is packed with calories) and make other adjustments, like eating skinless chicken.

Weight Watchers

Weight Watchers is based on a diet that mostly includes fruits, vegetables, eggs, skinless chicken breasts, fish, seafood, corn, beans, and peas. Other foods are allowed in limited quantities, including desserts, butter, pizza, hamburgers, fast food, cake, pie, ice cream, alcohol, and sugar-free soda. Before you get excited please note that these foods are consumed in very limited quantities. Weight Watchers uses a complicated point system and while it helps you control your portions, it doesn't help people who tire of the diet.

Advantages of the DASH Diet compared to other diets

With the exception of the Mediterranean diet, the DASH diet offers several key advantages:

- Unlike complicated point-counting schemes like Weight Watchers, the DASH diet is very easy to follow. Portioning out your servings is a snap.
- The DASH diet can be described as a careful application of "normal eating", so you're never going to feel totally deprived.
- The focus on limiting sodium and balancing sodium, potassium, magnesium, and calcium on the DASH diet makes it great for promoting cardiovascular health.

- Unlike radical diets such as Atkins or Keto, it doesn't require you to give up entire food groups for the rest of your conscious life.

- Unlike Paleo, it's not based on a made-up fad.

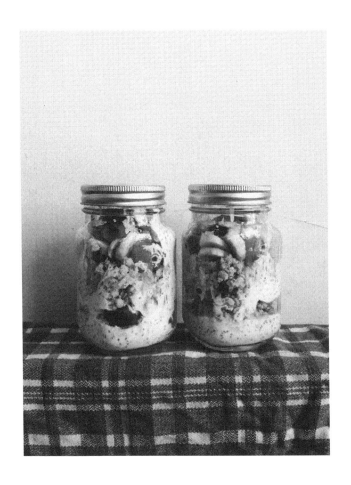

Chapter 3: The DASH Diet and Hypertension/High Blood Pressure

In the first chapter, we explained that high blood pressure can lead to multiple health problems. Let's explore this and its relation to the DASH diet in more detail.

Causes of High Blood Pressure

High blood pressure is one of the most serious health problems worldwide, with up to a billion people estimated to have high blood pressure. It's more acute in developed countries and when we examine possible causes of high blood pressure the reasons why become clear. In the United States, it's estimated that about 50 million people are suffering from high blood pressure. The actual number is unknown, and it's often called "the silent killer". The reason is that someone can appear to be completely healthy and yet have high blood pressure. Their body may look fine from the outside but internally it's being destroyed minute by minute.

As we mentioned earlier, in many cases, high blood pressure can be due to family history or genetics. However many environmental causes exist as well, and even if you have a family history your lifestyle choices may work against you or for you, however, the case may be. In other words, you might have the family history but if you don't smoke, maintain your weight, and exercise, you might avoid developing high blood pressure. Conversely, maybe you're relatively healthy even though you have a family history. Adopting an unhealthy lifestyle habit like smoking might tip you over the edge, leading to hypertension.

Some of the most common causes that have been identified include:

- Smoking: Cigarette smoking in particular, due to the fact people get more nicotine in their system, has been strongly identified as an environmental risk factor for developing high blood pressure.

- Weight gain/obesity: Not all overweight people have high blood pressure, but it's clear that being overweight significantly increases your risk of developing it. The heavier you get the higher the risk.

- Sedentary lifestyle: Exercise definitely counteracts hypertension. It helps keep the blood vessels flexible and responsive and helps keep the heart in shape. Someone who has cardiovascular fitness has a lower resting heart rate and their heart pumps with a healthier level of force, so the blood pressure is reduced as compared to what it would be otherwise. In contrast, people who don't exercise raise their risk of developing high blood pressure, especially if they have a family history.

- Race: African Americans are more prone to high blood pressure than other groups. However, bear in mind that all racial and ethnic groups have plenty of risk of high blood pressure and its victims include people of all races and from every country across the globe.

- Kidney disease: The kidneys are closely tied to the healthy maintenance of blood sugar. They help regulate the amount of fluid and salt in the body. When you are suffering from kidney disease they may not function as well, and this may lead to fluid and sodium retention which can cause high blood pressure.

- Age: Simply getting older raises risk, although we would never call high blood pressure "normal". However, as you get older things don't work as well (you knew that, right?). If your joints are stiffening you can bet your arteries are as well. So even though you may be reasonably healthy overall, simply getting older raises your risk of developing some level of high blood pressure. There is some debate about whether older people need to be put under the same standards as to what constitutes a diagnosis of hypertension or not, but a general rule applies. You're better off if your blood pressure is below 140/100.

- Nutritional deficiencies: By now you're an expert – nutritional deficiencies of potassium and magnesium can lead to the development of high blood pressure, along with other health problems like heart palpitations and muscle cramps.

- Excessive salt in the diet: We've reviewed this one already – salt causes your body to retain fluid and it promotes contraction of blood vessels, among other things.

The DASH diet provides an opportunity to address several items on this list. It reduces salt in the diet and addresses the nutritional deficiencies in potassium and magnesium. By consuming large amounts of fruits and vegetables along with a low-fat diet, you'll find that your risk of kidney disease drops as well. Controlling weight can also reduce the risks of developing high blood pressure.

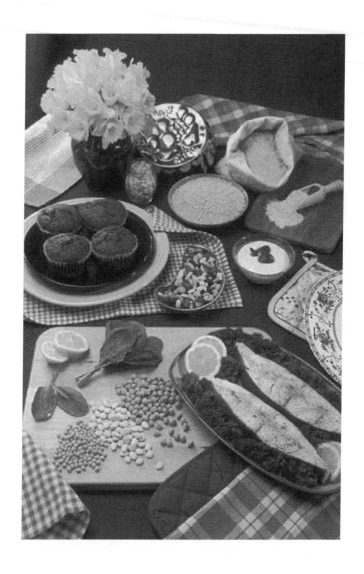

Chapter 4: The DASH Diet and Weight Loss

Normally people come to a diet hoping to achieve weight loss, and they look at getting the types of health benefits we've discussed so far as a nice side benefit. Usually, though, the DASH diet attracts people because they have been diagnosed with high blood pressure and their doctor has advised them to seek out the kind of lifestyle changes that the DASH diet offers. Regardless of the reasons why you came to the DASH diet, it can lead to substantial weight loss.

Effortless Weight Loss – How Does The DASH Diet Lead To Weight Loss

The DASH diet really isn't all that difficult to follow, because in many cases it simply mirrors what people normally eat already, with just a few adjustments. So instead of eating barbecued pork ribs, you eat a skinless barbecued chicken breast. You can have potato salad but use low-fat mayo. Adjustments like these really aren't all that difficult. Compare that to following a keto or Atkins diet, where you can't consume either barbecue sauce or eat potatoes. If your friend is having a July 4th party, they may not invite the keto dieters.

Portion Control

Remember Weight Watchers? It is basically designed for portion control – but it uses a complicated system. Most people don't want to mix accounting with eating, so weight watchers may still attract a lot of adherents but most people don't want to bother with that.

Other diets which fall into the low-fat category are based largely on counting calories. These types of diets can leave you feeling hungry and irritable. You may grow tired and mentally foggy since your body isn't getting enough to get by and you're not feeling full.

The DASH diet avoids calorie counting altogether. Instead, you simply follow the rules for the portion sizes outlined earlier, and then eat the number of items that the DASH food pyramid advises, provided you're not overindulging.

By specifying the maximum number of portions you can eat each day from each food group, you automatically get portion control without having to count calories or follow some complicated system. With an emphasis on low-calorie fruits and veggies and the consumption of a lot of fiber, you will also find that you fill yourself up to more easily. That way you never feel deprived, even though you're limiting portion sizes and numbers of portions consumed daily.

Limited Meat Consumption

We aren't advocating that people become vegan or vegetarian, although that is an option if you want to pursue it. But if you don't, one benefit of following the DASH diet is that it limits meat consumption. Meat in and of itself is not necessarily a bad thing, but remember that meat is dense in calories. In American society, people eat meat without any regard to portion size or even how many times per day they are eating it. Many people eat some kind of meat item for breakfast, lunch, and dinner. They might even snack on it.

The DASH diet forces you to think about how much meat you're eating, maybe for the very first time in your life. It also restricts servings of meat to 0-2 servings per day. That's a very easy rule to follow, and if you are following it for the first time you're going to be reducing the overall level of calories consumed per day on a practically autopilot level.

By cutting out the fat on beef and pork and skin on poultry, another source of calories can be eliminated. This also contributes to weight loss if you haven't been paying much attention to that up until this moment.

Eat Those Fruits and Veggies

What's one of the top benefits of eating several servings of spinach? Well, it's packed with all kinds of cancer-fighting nutrients and contains important minerals like potassium, but the advantage we're looking for here is that spinach is very low calorie. So you can eat a lot of spinach, broccoli, cauliflower, and other veggies and fill your stomach up without even thinking about it. The high fiber content of fruits and vegetables will help you feel satiated faster and reduce the temptation to eat a lot of meats and oils. The result of this is more weight loss.

Regulating Sweets

The DASH diet will help you get a handle on sweets and desserts – provided that you're truly committed to the diet, of course. First, the DASH diet tells you exactly how many servings to eat – five per week. Second, it has strict definitions of what counts as a "sweet" with the size of each serving specified in detail. Sure – you could cheat if you wanted – but then don't blame anyone else if you fail to reach your health and weight loss goals. However, if you follow the rules you will find the fact that the DASH diet allows some sweets will help you satisfy that old sweet tooth and secondly that you will be losing weight despite consuming five servings of sweets per week.

Final Thoughts

The DASH diet does not make pie in the sky promises about weight loss. Keto, Atkins, and many other diets do make such claims. The

DASH diet takes an entirely different approach, more akin to the turtle that wins the race rather than the hare, who has a good start in the race but loses.

The DASH diet, provided that you actually follow the rules, will generate slow but steady weight loss that will add up over time. Once you fully adjust to the rules to be followed on the diet you will find that it gets easier to follow as time goes on. When people get tired of avoiding pasta for the rest of their lives, and cheat on their deprivation diets you'll still be following yours since its not much different from what people would eat already, its just a healthier version of it with the relative proportions of foods changed around to promote more consumption of potassium and magnesium.

So the takeaways are:

- The DASH diet will help you lose weight.

- Expect weight loss to be gradual and slow, but steady. Don't look to lose 20 pounds in 10 days.

- The DASH diet is not a quick fix for weight loss – it's a lifestyle plan developed for overall health.

- The DASH diet won't just help you lose weight, it will help you keep your blood pressure under control as you age (and reduce it if you've developed hypertension), avoid diabetes, and many other health problems.

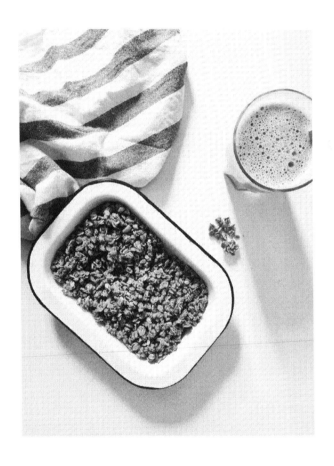

Chapter 5: What is Metabolic Syndrome?

We now turn our attention to one of the biggest health problems of the age: *metabolic syndrome.* In many cases, people who have high blood pressure are actually suffering from metabolic syndrome, and by following the DASH diet, they won't just cure their high blood pressure, they will reset their metabolism and eliminate metabolic syndrome from their lives.

Aside: Your Blood Lipids

Before we formally define metabolic syndrome, we need to review some basics about blood chemistry. The first area we need to review are blood lipids, which are basically the fats flowing around in your blood. Kind of gross, huh?

Don't worry, it's all perfectly natural and you need some level of blood fats. These fats take on a few different forms, some in combination with other molecules. This isn't a chemistry class so we aren't going to concern ourselves with the gory details, but we need to know what is in your blood and what the healthy levels of various components should be. Generally, we are concerned with the following:

- Total cholesterol
- LDL cholesterol
- HDL cholesterol
- Triglycerides

No doubt you've heard about total cholesterol already, it's been the focus of the medical community for many years. High total cholesterol is associated with increased risk of developing heart disease, and also with a higher risk of actually having a heart attack or stroke. In the United States, we measure cholesterol in milligrams of cholesterol per deciliter of blood, or mg/dL. A general rule of thumb is that a total cholesterol of 200 or less is considered low risk, while total cholesterol over 200 is considered elevated risk, with the risk significantly increasing for each 10 point increase in your total cholesterol. If you consistently show total cholesterol levels of 230 mg/dL or higher, your doctor may want to prescribe statin drugs, which lower cholesterol. Some doctors are more strict than others and will prescribe statins at even lower levels.

Total cholesterol is calculated the following way:

Total cholesterol = LDL Cholesterol + HDL Cholesterol + 0.20 * Triglycerides

You will often see your triglyceride level shown on your blood tests, what this means is that 20% of your triglyceride level is counted toward your total cholesterol number. Triglycerides are a type of fat that is carried around in your blood.

LDL means Low-Density Lipoprotein. A lipoprotein is a complicated molecule that is made of fat ("lipo") and proteins. Cholesterol is actually a substance transported through the blood by the LDL or HDL molecule.

LDL is called "bad cholesterol" because it can stick to the walls of your arteries. Over time, they become calcified and you develop fatty deposits and plaque, and the arteries can narrow, eventually causing a heart attack. The level of LDL cholesterol in your blood is directly related to the amount of saturated fat you eat per day. An easy way to lower your cholesterol if you're in the borderline range and your doctor isn't putting you on statins yet is to limit your consumption of saturated fats to 20 grams per day or less. Saturated fat is mostly found in animal products like beef and chicken skin, but it's in all animal products. Dairy and even fish also contain saturated fat. Coconut oil also contains a lot of saturated fat.

HDL is known as "good cholesterol". The reason is that HDL cholesterol is sort of a cleanup crew for the bloodstream. It picks up bad cholesterol, even cleaning it off the artery walls, and it brings it back to the liver. If you have a higher HDL cholesterol (greater than 45 mg/dL, about) then you're at lower risk of heart disease.

The ratio of total cholesterol to HDL can predict your risk of a heart attack. Generally, you're at lower risk of heart attack if:

Total Cholesterol/HDL < 5

So if someone has total cholesterol of 200 and an HDL cholesterol of 50, their ratio is:

200/50 = 4

This person is considered at low risk of having a heart attack over say, the next five years. Now suppose someone had total cholesterol of 220 and an HDL cholesterol of 35. Their ratio would be:

220/35 = 6.3

This person is at elevated risk for a heart attack. Their physician may put them on a statin and advise them to take up vigorous aerobic exercise.

While a ratio of less than five is desirable, a ratio of about 3 is considered ideal. While lowering total cholesterol can be achieved with statins, it's not really possible to raise HDL with any drugs. A better diet, losing weight, and exercise may raise your HDL.

Although cholesterol is portrayed as some kind of dangerous substance, it's actually a key component of the body. It's used to build and maintain cell membranes, and it's used to make important hormones in the body. You'd die without any cholesterol, and in fact, people with very low cholesterol (below 160) have higher rates of death from all causes.

Triglycerides are also important to measure. High triglycerides indicate a higher risk of heart attack and can cause other problems such as pancreatitis. The ratio of triglycerides to HDL cholesterol is a good indicator of heart attack risk, in fact, its better than looking at total cholesterol or even LDL "bad" cholesterol. If the ratio is 1 or less, you're considered to be at low risk of a heart attack. If it's greater than 1, then you're at higher risk.

High LDL cholesterol and a high triglyceride to HDL number not only indicate the risk of heart attack, but they are also a good way to evaluate the risk of stroke. To summarize, it's bad to have:

- High LDL cholesterol
- Low HDL cholesterol

- High triglycerides

Blood Sugar and Insulin

Now we move on from fat to sugar. Like cholesterol, your body needs some sugar in the blood. Without sugar, your brain can't power itself. And just like with cholesterol when your blood sugar goes too high, serious health problems will result.

The hormone insulin is closely tied to blood sugar. Basically, when you eat something your body begins to digest the carbohydrates in the food you ate. They are broken down into individual components called glucose, the simplest form of sugar or starch that there is. The glucose then enters your bloodstream.

The cells of your body need glucose for energy and your brain needs it to survive. However, the cells of the body aren't just going to suck up the glucose. They need a trigger, to be told to take it up. That trigger is provided by insulin. Think of insulin as a key fitting into the door of the cell and opening it, so that the glucose can go inside, and leave the bloodstream.

In a normal, healthy person, this process works fine. A healthy person could eat a plate of spaghetti, and about two hours later their blood sugar would be about 140 mg/dL (we measure blood sugar in the same units used to measure cholesterol).

However, some people begin to become resistant to insulin. Maybe you could think of it as the keys to the door wearing out, but over time, it takes more insulin to trigger the cells into taking up the sugar. The cells are said to become *insulin resistant.* As a result, the person is not getting the proper energy they need from the food, and their blood sugar goes higher than it does for a normal person after a meal. Eating that same plate of spaghetti, their blood sugar may go up to 180 mg/dL, or even 200 mg/dL. Blood sugar may stay elevated for longer periods of time. Eventually, the person will see blood sugar elevated even when fasting overnight. This is often the first sign that is caught by doctors that a patient may be pre-diabetic or diabetic.

The body isn't designed for elevated levels of glucose in the blood. High blood sugar will damage blood vessels, in particular, smaller blood vessels that supply organs and nerves. With reduced blood supply, over time various organs and nerves become damaged. This can cause kidney disease, vision problems, erectile dysfunction, and problems healing since the blood supply to peripheral wounds is compromised.

The pancreas, the organ that produces insulin, also suffers over time when someone has high blood sugars. In an attempt to compensate, it strains itself making more and more insulin. These things go together:

- A person who has high blood sugar
- Also has high levels of insulin
- And is insulin resistant

High glucose levels in the blood also damage your arteries. This leads to "hardening" of the arteries or atherosclerosis, which can lead to heart attack and stroke.

In addition, cancer cells love sugar. High blood sugar is associated with higher risks of cancer. In fact, diabetics have the higher risk for cancer as versus everyone else. Moreover, diabetics treated with the blood sugar controlling drug Metformin actually have a reduced risk of developing cancer.

Finally – Metabolic Syndrome

Now we are done with our science lectures, and we can come to the main topic of the chapter – metabolic syndrome. What is it? Well, we have started this book by observing that the DASH diet treats high blood pressure, but it turns out that high blood pressure and all the things discussed in this chapter are often closely related. A person that has all these problems is said to have metabolic syndrome because the cluster of health problems are related to a dysfunctional metabolic system that is related to problems digesting simple carbohydrates.

A diagnosis of metabolic syndrome involves having three or more of the following:

- Increased weight around the midsection.
- Elevated blood sugar and insulin resistance.
- High total cholesterol.

- High triglycerides.
- Low HDL cholesterol
- High blood pressure, above 135/85.

So now we've tied everything together – the problems that we've been describing, including high blood pressure, low HDL cholesterol and elevated blood sugars, seldom occur in isolation. If you look at the symptoms, it kind of looks like middle age in developed countries, especially in the United States. There is no question it's related to the unhealthy eating practices of the standard American diet.

The DASH Diet and Metabolic Syndrome

The DASH diet is a good diet for tackling metabolic syndrome. The diet is also designed to reduce blood pressure levels. Moreover, the moderate level of consumption of lean meats will help lower total cholesterol. Since over time, it will also lead to weight loss, the DASH diet will create a feedback loop that will lead to further improvement in all of these measures. In short, the DASH diet is made to order for metabolic syndrome. If the characteristics of metabolic syndrome sounds like you at all – then you should be considering the DASH diet among your options.

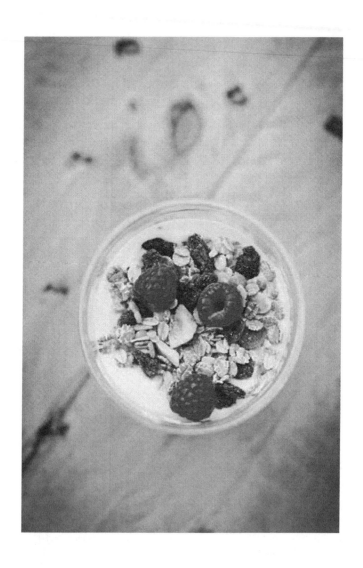

Chapter 6: The DASH Diet, Diabetes, and Heart Disease

The interesting thing about the "chronic" diseases of highly developed, western societies is that none of them occur in isolation. Consider that:

- Someone with diabetes is at elevated risk of heart disease and stroke.
- Someone with diabetes is at elevated risk of cancer.
- Someone with high blood pressure is at elevated risk of heart disease and stroke.
- Someone with diabetes is at elevated risk of high blood pressure.
- Someone with diabetes is at elevated risk of vision loss, nerve damage, and kidney disease.

- Someone with kidney disease is at elevated risk of developing high blood pressure.

It's pretty obvious that central casting would put diabetes in the lead role here. Or you could say that in the end, all roads lead to diabetes.

Doctors have tightened up the criteria for diabetes diagnosis, given the very serious nature of the disease. It's literally taking the lives of millions. In the United States, it's estimated that 100 million people either have diabetes or pre-diabetes. That is nearly 1/3 of the entire population, and a greater fraction of adults since young people are less likely to suffer from diabetes (however it's rising among young people, at alarming rates).

Let's look at the diagnostic criteria of diabetes and pre-diabetes. The first thing that doctors will look at is your fasting blood sugar levels.

Generally speaking, these are divided as follows, after 8-12 hours of fasting:

- Below 100 is considered normal.
- Greater than 100, but under 125 is considered "pre-diabetes".
- Over 125 on multiple occasions is considered full-blown diabetes.

What does pre-diabetes mean? Like pre-hypertension, it means that you may be able to reverse the condition through lifestyle changes. Of course, that means changes to diet and exercise. Weight loss is crucial here, people who are heavier tend to have more blood sugar problems. For a given individual, the more weight you gain the higher your risk of developing diabetes.

Doctors also take into account A1C, which is a test that looks at the hemoglobin in your blood to determine what your average blood sugar has been for the past 90 days. This test is actually more important than a fasting blood sugar test. Someone may not have a fasting blood sugar that is very high, but if their blood sugar goes really high after eating a meal and stays there it can cause problems. Those blood sugar spikes are the most damaging to blood vessels and tissues. It works for 90 days because red blood cells live for three months.

A1C is measured as a percentage. The normal range is considered to be between 4% and 5.6%. The A1C value corresponds to what the average blood sugar has been for the past 90 days. An A1C of 4% corresponds to an average blood sugar of 68 mg/dL, which is quite low. A level of 5.6% corresponds to an average blood sugar of roughly 112 mg/dL.

If your A1C ranges between 5.7% and 6.4%, which would be average blood sugar above 112 mg/dL to about 140 or so, you're considered at elevated risk for developing diabetes. A formal diabetes diagnosis sets in for an A1C level of 6.5% or higher.

Why DASH is good for diabetes or pre-diabetes

There are five main ways that a DASH diet can help people suffering from either pre-diabetes or diabetes. These are:

- A high fiber diet helps you digest more slowly.
- By consuming whole grains, you are less prone to blood sugar spikes – reducing the damage they cause.
- The emphasis on fruits and vegetables encourages the consumption of low glycemic foods (foods that are less prone to causing blood sugar spikes) and low-calorie foods, promoting better blood sugars and weight loss.

- Consuming lean meats will leave you feeling more satisfied and energetic, and less likely to eat lots of empty carbs to try and feel satiated.

- Milk and dairy, consumed on a regular basis, help you feel satiated.

Diabetes risk is also closely tied to weight. Since the portioning of the DASH diet with its an emphasis on less calorie dense foods encourages weight loss, it can help reduce your risk of developing diabetes. If you already have diabetes, it can help reduce your dependence on medications, and in some cases may even eliminate the need for medications.

DASH, Diabetes, and Heart Disease

Diabetics are at elevated risk for having a heart attack and stroke. Consider that nearly 70% of diabetics who are 65 and older die of heart attacks. In addition, some 16% will die of stroke.

Interestingly, even when blood sugar levels are controlled, diabetics remain at significantly elevated risk for heart disease. The reason harkens back to metabolic syndrome. Diabetics are also likely to have high blood pressure, high triglycerides, low HDL cholesterol, elevated total cholesterol, and they are more likely to be overweight.

The DASH Diet and Cholesterol

The DASH diet is a balanced diet that emphasizes high fiber, whole grains, and lean meats. Remember that saturated fat is made into LDL or bad cholesterol. By focusing on the consumption of lean meats, the DASH diet can lower LDL and total cholesterol in most people that follow it as directed. The American Heart Association recommends reducing the consumption of saturated fat to help control LDL and total cholesterol levels, hence reducing the risk of heart disease. The DASH diet does this very effectively. Since the DASH diet also encourages gradual, but sustainable weight loss, it will also reduce bad cholesterol and triglycerides in the blood through this route. If you lose about 10% of your body weight you will probably see improvement in your cholesterol and triglyceride numbers.

By eating wholesome foods, the DASH diet will also reduce the risk of blood sugar spikes and help control triglycerides. A healthy triglyceride level is 100 mg/dL or lower, while 150 mg/dL would be considered borderline.

By reducing blood sugar spikes, the DASH diet will not only help you avoid diabetes, but it will also help you avoid the kind of damage that high blood sugar causes to your blood vessels. This will not only reduce the risks of complication from diabetes like kidney disease, and vision loss, but will reduce the risk of developing problems like slow wound healing, that can lead to serious infections and even amputation.

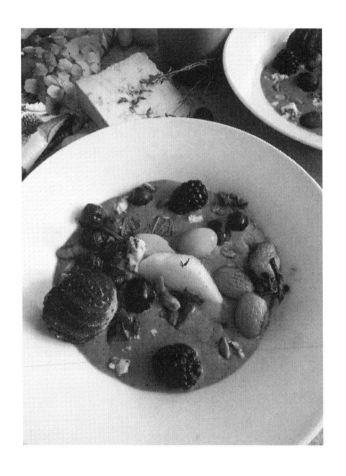

Chapter 7: The DASH Diet and Osteoporosis

The DASH diet wasn't designed with osteoporosis in mind, but it can help reduce the risk of developing it and help manage it if osteoporosis has already developed. This is a hugely beneficial side effect of the diet.

Osteoporosis is a huge public health issue. While not as many people suffer from it as is the case with diabetes, it's estimated that in the US alone there are 44 million adults with osteoporosis or low bone mass (although it's not called this, think of low bone mass as "pre-osteoporosis"). This is about 55 % of adults aged 50 and older.

Developing osteoporosis is a very serious health matter. Obviously, it can make it easier to break a bone. In particular, hip and spinal fractures are serious injuries that can happen to someone with osteoporosis. When a doctor is treating a patient with osteoporosis, the main goal is to prevent these kinds of fractures. A hip or spinal fracture can even lead to death, and its certainly going to lead to pain which may become chronic or disability.

One of the ways that osteoporosis can be treated or prevented – and acting at the stage of prevention is a far better proposition – is through diet. A balanced diet rich in calcium and vitamin D is recommended. While you can take supplements, it's best to get calcium through food (supplements of vitamin D3 may be warranted for most people, even those without osteoporosis).

Let's take a look at the foods that are recommended to help live a healthy lifestyle with osteoporosis or to prevent it in the first place:

- Green leafy vegetables including spinach, kale, mustard greens, and arugula.

- Foods rich in potassium such as oranges, bananas, tomatoes, potatoes, and sweet potatoes.

- Foods rich in vitamin C such as broccoli, Brussels sprouts, oranges.

- Fatty fish like mackerel and salmon.

- Canned fish with bones, including sardines and canned salmon.

- Dairy products such as low-fat milk, low-fat yogurt, and cheese.

Hopefully, you are looking over this list and thinking that looks familiar! The list is practically lifted from the DASH diet.

It turns out that many of the same foods that help the body naturally regulate blood pressure will also help prevent osteoporosis or help you manage it if you've already been diagnosed with it. These foods are rich in vitamin D, minerals like potassium and magnesium, vitamin k, and importantly calcium.

Another benefit of the DASH diet related to osteoporosis is that high consumption of salt can cause calcium and bone loss. Since the DASH diet's central premise is low sodium consumption it automatically combats this problem.

The inclusion of Dairy on the DASH diet is especially important. While many plant foods like spinach contain calcium, they also contain substances that inhibit the absorption of calcium from these foods. However, by consuming the daily recommended servings of milk, yogurt, and cheese, the DASH diet will give you adequate levels of calcium in your food that your body can easily utilize.

In fact, the ability of the DASH diet to help osteoporosis patients remain healthy is scientifically proven. Consider "The DASH diet and sodium reduction improve markers of bone turnover and calcium metabolism in adults."

The researchers found that following a DASH diet will reduce bone turnover. While a small level of bone turnover is normal, elevated bone turnover is associated with bone loss over time. Women are particularly susceptible because of the loss of estrogen that accompanies menopause increases bone turnover.

Researchers found that lowering sodium intake helps to reduce bone turnover by itself, but the effects are magnified when reduced sodium intake is incorporated into a wholesome diet that also incorporates the consumption of calcium and vitamin D. Most foods don't contain much vitamin D, but milk is fortified with it. What diet incorporates all of these food items, while also reducing sodium intake? The DASH diet is one such diet. In fact, it may be the only diet that brings all of these important dietary factors under a single roof.

More Nutrition per Meal

The key to the nutrition that you get from the DASH diet is its emphasis on consuming large amounts of fruits and vegetables. This means you'll be well-stocked on vitamins and minerals, and also when it comes to consuming phytonutrients and anti-oxidants that are associated with reduced risk of cancer. Moreover, the DASH diet aims for balance. With most meals, you'll be getting foods from every food group. That means that you'll get all the nutrients that there are in every single meal. Whole grains, for example, are packed with B-vitamins, while the fruit and veggies you eat with your meal will supply you with vitamins A & C. Meanwhile your required dairy will give you calcium and vitamin D.

DASH Diet and Cancer

High consumption of fruits and vegetables has been shown to reduce the risk of colorectal and other cancers, and the high fiber intake on the diet can also reduce the risk. Some studies have also shown that high amounts of consumption of red meat can lead to colorectal cancer. Since the DASH diet limits meat to moderate consumption levels and limits red meat consumption, even more, this is another way that the DASH diet can reduce the risk of colorectal cancer. High salt intake may also be related to certain cancers, and by reducing sodium intake the DASH diet significantly reduces these risks. While the DASH diet isn't as big on the consumption of nuts and seeds as say the Mediterranean diet, practitioners are advised to have one serving per day. Studies have shown that consumption of nuts on a regular basis may reduce the risk of breast cancer. They probably do this by reducing inflammation, and that may reduce the risk of other cancers as well. Since the DASH diet does favor nut consumption in moderation, it can lead to reduced levels of cancer that have been associated with nut consumption.

One study of colorectal cancer in Canada found that following the DASH diet reduced the risk of getting colorectal cancer by 33% as compared to those whose diet was the least like the DASH diet.

Some studies have shown that diets high in fats are linked with cancers. Since the DASH diet emphasizes a low-fat diet, this may reduce the risk of certain cancers – in particular, it may reduce the risk of pancreatic, breast, and colon cancer.

Since the DASH diet completely eliminates these foods, it's clear that the DASH diet will reduce the cancer risks associated with them.

DASH Diet and Stroke Risk

As reported by Harvard Health Review, patients who were tracked for 12 years who followed the DASH diet had a lower risk of stroke. In this case, the researchers were looking at a type of stroke which is called an ischemic stroke. This is due to a blood clot in the brain that is a result of fatty plaque buildup. The researchers speculated that the reduction in risk comes from the combination of lowered blood pressure combined with a healthier whole grain, lower fat diet. By consuming a lower fat diet the patients tracked in the study probably had less plaque in their arteries, which lowers the risk of stroke. The diet will also lessen the risk of ischemic (and hemorrhagic) stroke because of the simple fact that it lowers blood pressure. As we saw at the beginning of the book, high blood pressure is associated with a higher risk of both types of stroke.

Chapter 8: Summary of Health Benefit and Daily Macros

Let's review the health benefits of the DASH diet that we've discovered so far:

- The DASH diet is a low sodium diet. By lowering daily intake of sodium, the DASH diet helps lower blood pressure to healthy levels and reduces bone turnover, and hence reduces the risk of osteoporosis.

- The DASH diet is a low-fat diet. By reducing the intake of saturated fat in particular, the DASH diet will lower your LDL and total cholesterol levels, which in turn will reduce your risk of having a heart attack or stroke.

- The DASH diet is low fat, adequate protein, and high fiber emphasizing the whole grain and low glycemic foods. This helps to control or reduce the risk of diabetes.

- The DASH diet naturally forces you to control portions and portion sizes. Since it also consists of lower calorie foods, the DASH diet will help you lose weight. By losing weight you will reduce your risk of diabetes, heart disease, stroke, and cancer.

- The DASH diet is a balanced diet that includes the consumption of many green vegetables and dairy, providing good levels of calcium in your diet. This will reduce the risk of developing osteoporosis or help you manage it if you already have it.

- The DASH diet encourages the consumption of fish and seafood, which has been demonstrated to lower the risk of heart disease.

- Avoiding red meat may reduce the risk of certain cancers. In addition, the DASH diet eliminates processed meats from the diet which are associated with specific cancers as well.

- The DASH diet, by promoting healthy blood fats, keeping your blood pressure low and keeping your arteries clear, will improve brain function and improve mental health. Dementia has been associated with high blood pressure, and by controlling blood pressure the DASH diet can help reduce the risk of problems related to the brain that aren't directly the result of a stroke.

- The DASH diet limits the consumption of beans. While overall beans are healthy, beans contain chemicals that can increase bone loss. You can reduce the chemicals by soaking the beans and rinsing before cooking.

We have avoided discussions of calories because unlike weight watchers or other low-fat diets, the DASH diet is not built around the idea of counting your calories and trying to starve yourself into health. That said, simply following the advice of the DASH diet – eating the correct portion sizes and the recommended number of daily portions from each food group found on the DASH diet pyramid, you will find yourself naturally limiting the total number of calories consumed. Generally, calories consumed on the DASH diet can range between 1,600 to 3,000 calories per day, depending on your body size. The rule of thumb to use here simply is to follow the recommendations for portions and portion sizes and eats until you're satiated.

Now let's have a look at the recommended macro consumption for a so-called "standard" dietary intake, which is taken to be 2,000 calories per day.

- Sodium: up to 2,300 mg per day.

- Potassium: At least 3,500 mg per day, up to 4,700 mg per day.

- Magnesium: At least 500 mg per day.

- Calcium: At least 1,250 mg per day.

- Carbohydrates: About 55% of daily calorie intake.

- Protein: About 18% of daily calorie intake.

- Fat: About 27% of daily calorie intake.

- Saturated fat: About 6-10% of daily calorie intake.

- Dietary fiber: 30 grams per day.

The Low Sodium Option

For those with more intractable blood pressure problems that don't respond well to the DASH diet, there is a lower sodium version of the diet that should be considered. This version of the diet limits the dietary intake of sodium to 1,500 mg per day. All other food items are consumed in the amounts shown in the above listing. Be sure to discuss this with your doctor.

Estimating your needed calories

According to the national institutes of health, an average woman aged 19-30 will need 2,000 calories per day if she is sedentary. If she is moderately active, she may need up to 2,200 calories per day. Active women will need up to 2,400 calories. For those aged 31-50, needed calories are about 200 per day lower in all categories. For a sedentary man, aged 19-30, the daily caloric intake is 2,400 calories. A moderately active man will require between 2,600-2,800 calories, while an active man will need 3,000 calories per day. As men enter the age groups 31-50 and 51+, daily caloric needs for all categories drop about 200 calories per day. Sedentary is defined as someone who only does light physical activity as part of their daily routine. In other words, they don't exercise. A moderately active person is defined as someone who engages in walking, maybe 1.5-3 miles per day. Active means a person who walks longer distances or who engages in more vigorous exercise like running.

The National Institutes of Health has worked out detailed daily servings for the DASH diet broken down by daily required calories. For example, a woman who is 35 and sedentary will consume 6 servings of grains per day, while an active woman who is 25 would need to consume 8-10 servings per day.

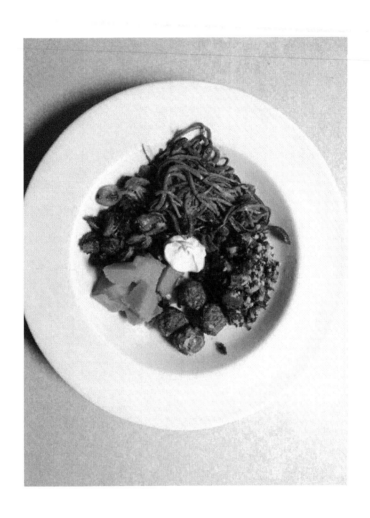

Chapter 9: Myths about the DASH Diet

Like any dietary regimen, many myths swirl around the DASH diet. Let's take some time to examine what they are and correct any misconceptions that you may still have about the diet.

The DASH Diet is a no-salt diet

Nothing could be further from the truth. In fact, while many believe this convenient myth, it can only be described as absurd. First of all, it would be virtually impossible to eat a no-salt or no-sodium diet. Almost every food contains at least a little bit of sodium.

Second, the diet doesn't recommend that you stop sodium intake, it recommends that you reduce sodium intake. The average American consumes around 3,500 mg per day. Remember that is average! That means that lots of people are consuming a lot more than 3,500 mg per day. We've seen that high sodium intake is associated with high blood pressure, fluid retention, and even osteoporosis.

The DASH diet has specific recommendations that you consume 2,300 mg of sodium per day. This is more than enough sodium and its still a large fraction of the sodium that is consumed by the average person (to wit: 66% or about 2/3). Does a diet that recommends that you consume 2/3 of the amount of sodium the average person consumes sound like a no-salt diet?

Even the low sodium version – which is not going to be followed by most people anyway – allows you to consume 1,500 mg of sodium per day.

The DASH Diet is a High Blood Pressure Diet

This one is tricky because there is actually some truth to it. Yes, the DASH diet was originally developed to treat high blood pressure using diet. However, we've seen the long list of health benefits the DASH diet provides, including weight loss. The bottom line is that the DASH diet is an all-around healthy diet of the kind that medical professionals have been recommending for decades, even if they weren't doing so in the detailed specifics. The DASH diet not only keeps blood pressure under control, but it also helps to lose weight and helps you avoid a wide range of health problems. As such it can be described as an all-around healthy approach toward nutrition. Any person can benefit from this, not just folks that suffer from high blood pressure. Moreover, you may not suffer from high blood pressure now, but you could develop it as you age. The DASH diet will reduce the risk of that happening.

The DASH Diet is Complicated and Hard to Follow

Nothing could be further from the truth. The rules that the diet is based on are actually probably the simplest rules in the entire world of diet and nutrition. Rather than running around with cards, counting every little bit up and weighing things on scales, you simply follow the portion rules (1 slice of bread, a fruit, a vegetable, lean meat and a cup of milk, etc.) to determine what to eat. There is nothing complicated about it.

It's hard to incorporate the DASH diet with friends and Family

Again, this is another myth that simply isn't true. Think about what kinds of foods are on the DASH diet in general terms:

- Fruit
- Veggies
- Meat
- Dairy
- Beans and nuts

Hmm, does that list look at all familiar? It's basically what most people eat. So there should not be a problem fitting the DASH diet in with your family or even your friends, who may think you are nuts if you start lecturing them about DASH. Our advice is shown them with the health benefits and weight loss you achieve while following the DASH diet.

You can't eat out on the DASH Diet

Actually, the DASH diet is one of the easiest diets that you can follow when it comes to incorporating it with eating out. You can easily ask the waiter to have the cook make a low salt version of a dish you order in a restaurant.

Simply avoiding the urge to add salt to your meal when eating out goes a long way towards keeping yourself on the diet. Compare that to someone on a specialized diet that bans entire food groups, who may find they can hardly eat out anywhere and coming to an agreement with friends is difficult. When the bread comes out, you can have a slice while your friend on "keto" is squirming in their seat. You can always request low-fat versions of salad dressings. Even fast food is easier to accommodate on the DASH diet – just skip the salty French fries.

The DASH Diet is Expensive

In fact, the DASH diet may reduce your food bill. Remember that the DASH diet has you eating meat, but only twice a day and the recommendation is actually 0-2 times per day. What's more expensive – oatmeal or rib eye steak? By keeping your meat consumption moderate you save space in your refrigerator and reduce your food bill. In the past, while whole grain bread and pasta were expensive and even hard to find, now many lower cost varieties are available.

The DASH Diet will leave you unsatisfied

As we've emphasized, the DASH diet is not one that is based on deprivation. You should eat your required calorie intake on the DASH diet. Also, it incorporates whole grains, fruits, and vegetables that will fill you up and help you get satisfied without overdoing it on calories. While other diets leave you counting every last calorie and gram, you eat on DASH until you're satisfied as long as you're not exceeding the recommended daily portions. Try it and you'll see that this is more than adequate for leaving you feeling satisfied.

The DASH diet means giving up favorite foods

This is a problem – when you're trying Atkins or keto. Remember those diets limit carbohydrates to such paltry levels you probably overreach by simply breathing. The DASH diet is different – rather than giving up pasta for the rest of your life or steak, instead, you consume your food in moderation. The DASH diet is a diet of moderation, not deprivation.

The DASH Diet has unpleasant side effects

Have you heard about these nutty people following the "carnivore" diet? It's a *zero carb* diet. In other words, all you eat is meat and eggs. People that start his diet develop major digestive complications because they get no fiber.

Well, the DASH diet isn't like that. With DASH, you are simply following a normal diet, but just doing it in moderation. You're not going to get constipated or have trouble sleeping by cutting your salt back and eating lean cuts of meat.

Well, we hope that our discussion of the major myths and misconceptions about the DASH diet has put your mind at ease if you shared any of these beliefs about the diet.

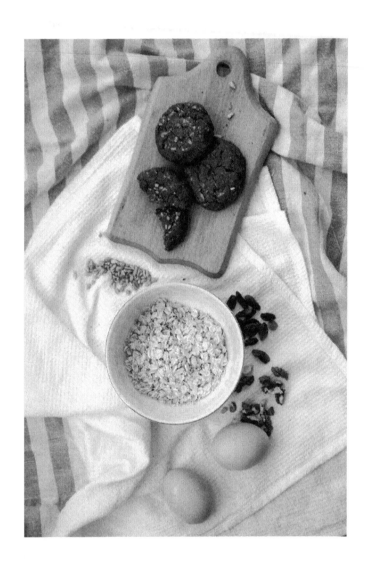

Chapter 10: The DASH Diet Food List

Now let's take a deep dive into foods you can eat and foods you should either consume in moderation or avoid completely while following the DASH diet. Remember, the starting point of the DASH diet is to limit sodium consumption. If this is your first time on the DASH diet, it's advised that you follow the standard DASH diet which limits sodium consumption to 2,300 mg per day. To be honest, you don't need to be completely religious about it. If you end up eating 2,500 mg of sodium per day you're still OK, and if you eat 2,200 one day and 2,800 the next you're fine too, if your average for the entire week comes in around 2,300-2,500 mg per day. As long as you're staying well below the average American who is consuming 3,400 mg per day of sodium, you're probably doing well at meeting your overall goals.

If you are going on this diet because of high blood pressure, and you find that hitting close to the 2,300 mg average but not seeing any results, then you can try the low sodium version of the diet. This limits sodium intake to 1,500 mg per day. Be sure to discuss these issues with your doctor before doing so.

Remember that the main components of the DASH diet are fruits and vegetables, whole grains, lean meats, and low-fat dairy. The DASH diet doesn't worry about calorie counting or weighing food, just refer back to the DASH diet food pyramid to get portion counts and sizes. We're going to look at a few items in detail since the DASH diet is so focused on getting the right amounts of potassium, sodium, magnesium, and calcium, it helps to have some awareness of what some foods actually contain.

Fruits

Fruits tend to contain large amounts of potassium and magnesium and very low sodium. As a result, they play a central role in the DASH diet. For example, let's look at the nutrition content of a medium sized apple:

- Calories: 95
- Sodium: 2 mg
- Potassium: 195 mg
- Magnesium: 2% of the daily value
- Calcium: 1% of the daily value

We picked an apple as our first example on purpose. You remember that in Japan, it was noticed that people in regions where large amounts of apples were consumed had much lower rates of stroke. By looking at the nutrition facts of an apple, we see that there is virtually no sodium in an apple at all, but a fair amount of potassium. So eating an apple a day really does keep the doctor away, in the sense that it's going to help rebalance your electrolytes by adding potassium practically all by itself. Let's check the nutrition facts for a large orange:

- Calories: 87
- Sodium: 0 mg
- Potassium: 333 mg
- Magnesium: 4% of the daily value
- Calcium: 7% of the daily value

Orange is even better for the DASH diet than an apple – it's got a lot more potassium and no sodium at all while giving us slightly higher amounts of calcium and magnesium.

The DASH diet was developed way back in 1992, during a time when fat was the enemy. If you've been paying attention you've probably noticed that the attitude about fat is shifting. When it comes to certain types of fat, like the omega-3 oils in fish and the monounsaturated fat in olive oil, the attitude has completely transformed and now these types of fats are viewed not only as healthy but perhaps as vital to good health, in particular for the cardiovascular system.

With that in mind, although it's not generally discussed within the context of the DASH diet – I would like to introduce you to the avocado. Those who are interested in following the "Mediterranean" version of the DASH diet will certainly be interested in avocados. Like olive oil, avocado oil is primarily monounsaturated fat, which is believed to reduce inflammation. The only issue with avocados is to be aware of the calorie content – since they are a fat based fruit they do pack more calories than most fruits. A suggestion is to eat a ½ of an avocado instead of a whole one, and of course, there is wide variation in size so you can reap the benefits while opting for smaller avocados with fewer calories. Let's look at the nutritional content of a medium-sized avocado:

- Calories: 332
- Fat: 29 grams (20 g is monounsaturated fat)
- Sodium: 14 mg
- Potassium: 975 mg
- Magnesium: 14% of the daily value
- Calcium: 2% of the daily value

If you'll take a close look, you'll notice that avocados are PACKING in potassium. If you're shooting for 4,700 mg of potassium per day, as recommended by the DASH diet, then avocado is a good start. Moreover, avocados also contain 14% of daily recommended magnesium. Avocados are also loaded with dietary fiber. One avocado provides 40% of the fiber you need each day.

While the DASH diet allows the consumption of frozen and dried fruits, you may think carefully about consuming these foods. This issue comes up because once again the DASH diet was originally developed in 1992. In a nutritional sense, it almost seems like the dark ages. At that time there wasn't the awareness of the problems with sugar consumption that there is now. The problem with frozen and dried fruit is that they contain concentrated sugar. You will want to avoid sugar and make sure you consume the whole fruit with all the fiber. The fiber helps slow digestion and reduces blood sugar spikes, along with all the harm that comes with them. For that reason, although fruit juice is permitted daily on the DASH diet, we recommend only consuming it in moderation, if at all. This advice is especially important for people who have pre-diabetes or who are diabetic. In that case, you're far better off eating an avocado than you are drinking orange juice, or indulging in dried fruit snacks.

Peach is also an excellent choice for fruit. It's low calorie and high potassium.

- Calories: 59
- Sodium: 0 mg
- Potassium: 285 mg
- Magnesium: 3% of daily value
- Calcium: 0% of daily value

Here is a complete list of fruits you can choose from to round out your first month on the DASH diet:

- Apple
- Avocado
- Banana
- Blackberries
- Blueberries
- Cantaloupe
- Cherries
- Dates
- Grapes
- Kiwi
- Mango

- Nectarines
- Oranges
- Peach
- Raspberries
- Strawberries
- Tomatoes

Yes, don't forget that tomatoes are fruits even though they kind of seem like vegetables. Berries are an excellent choice because they are packed with nutrients but have a low sugar content and glycemic index when compared to most fruits. We could list far more fruits than we have here, but we're going to limit our food lists because we want to keep things as simple as possible for people starting out with the DASH diet.

Vegetables

Remember that fruits and vegetables from the base of the DASH diet pyramid and that you should be consuming 4-5 servings of each.

Vegetables are great because other than starchy vegetables, they provide a lot of nutrients including vital minerals and they pack them in with hardly any calories. A serving of broccoli has a mere 50 calories while packing in the nutrition.

- Calories: 50
- Sodium: 49 mg
- Potassium: 468 mg
- Magnesium: 7% of daily value
- Calcium: 7% of daily value

A cup of cauliflower is also a good choice:

- Calories: 27
- Sodium: 32 mg
- Potassium: 320 mg
- Magnesium: 4% of the daily value
- Calcium: 2% of the daily value

Now let's take a look at a one cup serving of spinach.

- Calories: 7
- Sodium: 2 mg
- Potassium: 167 mg
- Magnesium: 5% of daily value
- Calcium: 2.4% of daily value

With hardly any calories, a cup of spinach is a good way to beef up your potassium. Now let's look at a carrot.

- Calories: 25
- Sodium: 42 mg
- Potassium: 195 mg
- Magnesium: 1% of daily value
- Calcium: 2% of daily value

Keep in mind that carrots do contain about 3 grams of sugar.

Now let's look at a couple of starchy vegetables. We'll look at a medium-sized ordinary potato first:

- Calories: 163
- Sodium: 13 mg
- Potassium: 897 mg
- Magnesium: 12% of the daily value
- Calcium: 2% of the daily value

People don't tend to think of plain potatoes as nutritious, but you can see they pack a lot more than starch. You also get 70% of your daily requirements for vitamin C from a potato. And this is a plain, white potato – the kind you'd use for baking. Maybe potato chips are more nutritious than we thought... if you decide to enjoy a baked potato be sure to season with something other than salt. You can also try using a little olive oil instead of slathering on butter.

What about sweet potatoes? Let's check:

- Calories: 114
- Sodium: 73 mg
- Potassium: 448 mg
- Magnesium: 8% of the daily value
- Calcium: 4% of the daily value

A sweet potato only provides 7% of vitamin C, but it does provide 377% of vitamin A. Comparing, ordinary potatoes are just as nutritious if not more so than sweet potatoes (with the exception of vitamin A). It's funny that many people perceive sweet potatoes to be healthy and ordinary potatoes to be practically junk food, only providing starch.

You may be noticing that vegetables provide more sodium than fruits. However, they also contain a lot more potassium and magnesium. And its all about balance.

Here is our suggested list of vegetables for your first month on the DASH diet:

- Artichoke hearts
- Arugula
- Asparagus
- Brussels sprouts
- Cabbage
- Carrots
- Celery
- Kale
- Mustard greens
- Onions
- Peppers
- Potatoes
- Spinach
- Spring mix and other lettuce
- Sweet potatoes
- Turnips

Whole Grains

Now we move on to grains, which includes bread, cereals, pasta, and rice. You're allowed 7-8 servings per day, but they should be whole grains. So what does that mean exactly?

Grains are essentially grasses, and you're eating the seeds. The seed contains three parts: the germ, the endosperm, and the bran. A food item made out of whole grains contains all three parts of the seed. In contrast, a refined grain contains only the endosperm. White bread, white flour, regular pasta, and white rice are examples of refined grains. While following the DASH diet you should not consume these types of food. They digest faster and hence raise blood sugar more, and you might as well think of them as nothing more than sugar.

Whole grains are divided into cereals and pseudo-cereals. Examples of cereals include wheat, corn, oats, rye, rice, and millet. Examples of pseudo-cereals are Buckwheat, Chia, and Quinoa.

Whole grains are rich in dietary fiber and also packed with nutrition including protein but also the minerals we seek including potassium and magnesium. They also contain lots of B-vitamins.

When purchasing grain products, make sure they are truly whole grain. Some snack products may be acceptable but make sure they are whole grain, are a reduced sodium variety, and they don't contain any harmful trans fats. Avoid sourdough bread and French bread. A partial list of grains to get for your first month includes:

- Bread of any variety provided it's whole grain. You can include rye as well.
- Breakfast cereals provided that they are whole grain and contain no added sugars.

- Brown rice.

- Buckwheat.

- Corn/Maize. Some people think of corn as a vegetable, it's a grain, so it doesn't count toward your required servings of veggies.

- Oats and oat bran.

- Pasta, as long as its whole grain. Some "white" pasta are available that are whole grain but read labels carefully.

- Quinoa.

- Rye bread (if you have a taste for it).

- Wild rice.

Dairy

Dairy is consumed daily but is to be consumed in moderation as compared to fruits, vegetables, and whole grains. You can have 2-3 servings of dairy per day. Generally, dairy is limited to:

- Milk
- Yogurt

- Cheese

The following items are to be avoided: cream, half-and-half, sour cream, butter, and buttermilk. The original DASH diet advised patients to consume low-fat varieties of dairy. However, recent studies have shown that people have success on the DASH diet even when consuming full-fat versions of dairy products like whole milk and regular cheese. In fact, they actually do better in some respects. It's been shown that they achieve better blood lipid values including total cholesterol, LDL or bad cholesterol, HDL or good cholesterol, and triglycerides. Which option you pursue is up to you, if you are having problems with your blood lipids you might at least want to try going with the full-fat versions of dairy for about a month or two and see how it affects your numbers. Since you only eat 2-3 servings per day, it's not going to throw off the rest of your diet calorie wise.

Here is the nutrition for a cup of whole milk:

- Calories: 148
- Sodium: 105 mg
- Potassium: 322 mg
- Magnesium: 6% of the daily value
- Calcium: 27% of the daily value

For a cup of yogurt, we have:

- Calories: 100
- Sodium: 61 mg
- Potassium: 240 mg
- Magnesium: 4% of the daily value
- Calcium: 18% of the daily value

While dairy products do contain significant amounts of sodium, they are perfectly healthy since they contain more potassium. They also provide important calcium and some magnesium as well. If osteoporosis is an issue that you're worried about, having a cup of milk and a serving of yogurt each day should be an important part of your diet. In fact, you should probably consume the fully allowed 3 portions, either by adding some cheese or a second serving of milk or yogurt if that describes your situation.

Meat

When it comes to meat, the DASH diet is fairly flexible but it does take the perspective of a low-fat diet. As a result, low-fat cuts of meat and poultry without skin are the order of the day. Since fish fat is deemed healthy, you can eat a serving of fatty fish without worrying about it.

A serving size of meat is 3 oz, but to be that strict all the time is probably beyond most people. So you might aim for between 3-5 oz servings. When craving foods like hamburger or sausage, you can still enjoy them if you look for low-fat alternatives made out of meats like turkey and chicken.

Poultry should be consumed without the skin. That means chicken wings are out, but skinless chicken breast and skinless chicken thighs are in. Turkey legs and thighs have too much fat when it comes to turkey you should stick to the skinless breast. Duck is a popular poultry item, but its best avoided on the DASH diet because duck has a high-fat content relative to chicken and turkey.

Lean cuts of beef can be enjoyed on a moderate basis. That means don't eat beef every day. There is no specific recommendation, but you should probably aim for once a week or less. When selecting beef, aim for lean cuts like sirloin. Ground beef can be consumed on occasion provided that you get the lowest fat variety that is available (shoot for 96%). Pork sausage should be avoided. When consuming other pork products, avoid ribs and aim for lean pork loins, or pork chops that have been trimmed of fat. Pork is considered a "red meat" by many experts, even though the pork industry used to try selling itself as the "other white meat".

For beef, you should select sirloin, chuck shoulder, top loin, round steaks, and roasts. Fatty cuts like prime rib, rib eye, porterhouse, t-bone, and new york strip should be avoided.

Exotic meats can find their way on the DASH diet menu to make your meals more interesting and varied. For example, consider elk which is available in stores like Whole Foods and Sprouts. Elk is similar to beef in taste and texture (we are talking farm-raised elk here) but its extremely lean. Many cuts of elk steak are only 3% fat.

Other exotic meats – of the farm-raised variety – you can consider include kangaroo and ostrich. These are also both red meat and extremely lean.

Processed meats should be avoided at all cost. So you should not be consuming salami, pepperoni, hot dogs, or even bacon, even if they are low-fat varieties. The main reason is that you must avoid the high sodium content of these meats.

When it comes to fish, you can consume virtually everything as long as you don't overdo the portions. Feel free to eat salmon, tuna, sardines, mackerel, swordfish, and trout to your desired level, up to 2 servings per day. You can also consume lean fish like cod and sole provided that it's not breaded unless the coating is made from whole grain flour. The health benefits of fish oil, when consumed in whole fish, are indisputable. The only fish that is really prohibited are canned anchovies and salted cod. Anchovies as you probably know are packed in salt and on a diet that is based on low sodium intake, anchovies don't make the cut.

Other types of seafood, being the leanest proteins on the planet, are definitely acceptable on the DASH diet. This includes shrimp, scallops, oysters, crab, and lobster. However, remember that your consumption of "butter" is limited to margarine and in small amounts. If you do eat lobster with butter (use a substitute like margarine, we are speaking colloquially here) make sure you know how much you're using. No doubt it's going to exceed the specified amounts allowed by the DASH diet per day – but you could make up for it the following day by consuming reduced servings from the oil, salad dressing, and mayo category.

Beans, Nuts, and Seeds

Next up we have the beans, nuts, and seeds category. If you're seeking out a low-fat diet, beans are often highly recommended because they have low fat, they are high-quality protein, and they have lots of fiber. If you're a vegan or vegetarian you can substitute them for the 0-2 servings of meat per day. However, if you're a meat eater you'll be limiting your servings of beans, nuts, and seeds, to one serving per day. This category also includes so-called "legumes" such as lentils, peas, and soybeans. Peanuts are also technically a legume, although most of us think of them as nuts.

You have the option of selecting nuts or seeds for your daily serving. Nuts and seeds have high-fat content, which is why they aren't recommended in large amounts. However, note that nuts have lots of healthy monounsaturated fat and also contain large amounts of potassium and magnesium.

It's understandable why nuts and seeds are limited to one serving daily since they contain a lot of fat and therefore they're calorie dense.

However, it's not really clear why the designers of the DASH diet would limit the consumption of beans. Beans are rich in certain vitamins, provide a practically zero fat source of protein, and also contain large amounts of needed dietary fiber. What's not to love about beans in the context of a healthy diet? In our view, you can increase bean consumption if you substitute it for meat. Studies show that people who eat nuts on a daily basis have significantly reduced risk of heart disease. So it makes more sense to eat a serving of nuts once per day and then when you want to eat beans, substitute them for a serving of meat.

Salad Dressing, Oils, and Mayo

The DASH diet is very restrictive when it comes to these items. You're only allowed 2-3 servings per day. Examples include:

- Canola oil
- Olive oil

- Mayo
- Low-fat or fat-free salad dressings
- Soft margarine, but consider smart balance which is hard but a very healthy alternative.

Sweets

Finally, we come to the topic of sweets. As we discussed earlier, "sweets" in the DASH diet might not meet your concept of sweets. They aren't talking about cake, pie, and ice cream, although they do allow small amounts of sugar, honey, and syrup. For the DASH dieter, a sweet consists of frozen yogurt or a serving of yogurt with fruit. It's not entirely clear why frozen yogurt is permitted while ice cream is not. Our take is you can eat certain varieties of ice cream – using the limited five serving per week guide. But be careful and read labels. Let's compare the nutrition for a ½ cup serving of frozen yogurt to a ½ cup serving of vanilla ice cream. According to a search on nutrition facts on Google, for the yogurt we have:

- Calories: 114
- Fat grams: 4
- Sugar: 17

For vanilla ice cream we find:

- Calories: 137
- Fat grams: 7
- Sugar: 14

Since we're only having at most five servings per week, that extra 23 calories and 3 grams of fat from vanilla ice cream are not going to matter at all. The increased fat in the vanilla ice cream is matched by more sugar in the yogurt. You could argue that you should have low-fat yogurt, but you can get low-fat vanilla ice cream as well. So in our view, as long as you carefully measure your servings, and only consume up to five servings per week, some real ice cream isn't going to throw off your diet.

And if you think it is, then but the ice cream for a time and see if things improve.

Alcohol

Alcohol is not explicitly discussed on the DASH diet, but it's so important we better mention it for those readers who are adults and like to drink. The general thought is that alcohol can be consumed in moderation while following the DASH diet. That means for men, 2-3 drinks per day and for women 1-2 drinks per day. You need to be aware that alcohol does add extra calories, especially if you're imbibing mixed drinks that can be loaded up with sugar, syrups, and cream. It's best to stick to straight liquor or even better beer and wine. While the DASH diet is not a calorie counting diet, you need to have some awareness if you drink alcohol. That means cutting some calories somewhere else. You might, for example, consider wine as a serving of fruit. And quite frankly, it is. Let's look at the nutrition of red wine:

- Calories: 125
- Sodium: 6 mg
- Potassium: 187 mg
- Magnesium: 4% of the daily value
- Calcium: 1% of the daily value

That nutrition profile isn't much different from that seen for many fruits, and that really isn't surprising since wine is made out of grapes, but I doubt that many readers have thought of drinking wine to get some extra potassium.

Beer also provides some potassium, but it also contains more sodium. It also provides a small amount of magnesium. Beer is more starchy, so if you are going to drink beer, you might consider substituting it for one serving of grains. Calling beer a vegetable might be too much of a stretch.

One concern regarding alcohol is that consuming alcohol can increase blood pressure in some people. You'll need to check this out for yourself and see if you're sensitive to that.

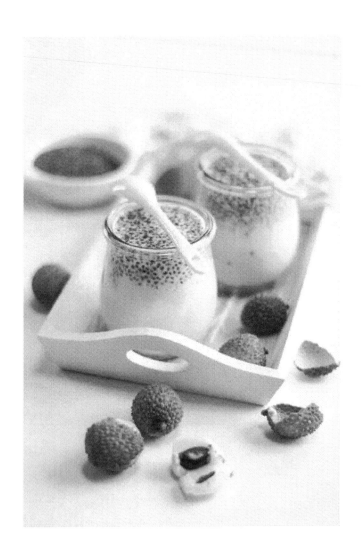

Chapter 11: Foods to Avoid on the DASH Diet

Although we've discussed many foods to avoid, we thought for the sake of having a reference we'll gather them here. When it comes to fruits and vegetables, there are no foods that are prohibited. So we'll start with grains.

Prohibited grains:

- White bread.
- White rice.
- White pasta.
- White, refined flour.
- White hamburger buns and hot dog rolls.
- Sourdough bread.
- French bread.
- Any cereal with added sugar.

- Breakfast "cereals" made from refined grains and flour.
- Any snacks containing sugar.
- Any snacks that have high sodium content (example – Triscuits may be whole grain, but they have a lot of salt. Get a low sodium variety).
- Any snacks that contain trans fats.

Next, let's look at dairy. Technically speaking, you can only consume low-fat varieties of milk, yogurt, and cheese. However, as we mentioned studies show that consuming the whole fat varieties makes no difference in outcomes, and in fact provides better outcomes, at least in some people.

However, there are some dairy products to avoid:

- Butter and ghee

- Heavy cream
- Whipped cream
- Half-and-Half
- Buttermilk
- Egg nog

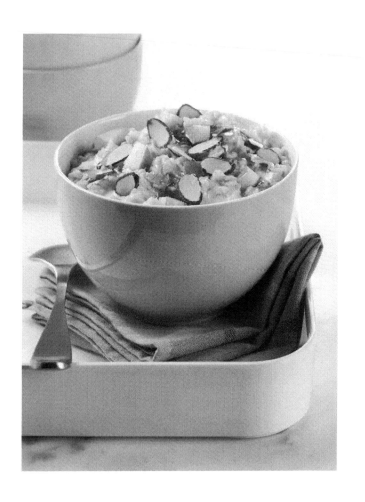

172

Chapter 12: Combining Exercise with the DASH Diet

Exercise forms an important component of your health. However, it's important to realize that for most of us exercise is not going to lead to weight loss. The bottom line is that to get weight loss from exercise, you'd have to spend all day engaged in physical activity and train at a high level. Most of us don't have the time for that, and diet is far more effective than exercise when it comes to weight loss anyway.

When you engage in a cardiovascular exercise which is extremely strenuous, you can even scar the heart and raise the body's level of inflammation. It's hard to believe but it's true – people who engage in high-intensity exercise are actually at elevated risk of a heart attack. It seems paradoxical until you realize that a heart attack can also be caused by increased inflammation.

For these reasons, the DASH dieter should focus on moderate exercise. The definition of moderate exercise is not entirely rigorous, we'll investigate a few different ways that you can incorporate exercise into your daily routines. However, remember that you're not exercising for the purpose of losing weight. Instead, the DASH dieter exercises for the purpose of maintaining general good health.

That said, when it comes to blood pressure, as we'll see in a moment, the effects of the DASH diet are enhanced by regular aerobic exercise.

Benefits of Aerobic Exercise

We'll investigate the different options that are available when it comes to exercise in a moment. For now, let's examine some of the health benefits.

Exercise, lowers the overall risk of death. The risk of death decreases for all causes – indicating that exercise reduces the risk of death from cancer, cardiovascular disease, kidney disease, and possibly many others. When it comes to heart disease and stroke, the benefits are immediately obvious and clear.

Regular exercise will help you maintain healthy blood levels. Even if you already have hypertension, you should get out there and get moving so that your health problems don't get any worse, and might possibly improve. One thing that exercise does that may help some mildly hypertensive patients, is it causes your blood vessels to widen, as they need to carry extra blood to the large muscle groups to keep them adequately supplied during physical activity. This helps your blood vessels stay in shape, remaining supple and pliant, rather than stiff and brittle. That means they will better respond to changes in blood pressure and stress.

Aerobic exercise can raise your HDL level and lower LDL cholesterol. By engaging in regular aerobic exercise, you can lower the chanced of acquiring heart disease by improving your blood lipids.

In addition to benefits that affect blood lipids, exercise will strengthen your heart. Why? Because when you're engaged in physical activity, your blood pressure goes up and the heart has to work harder to pump blood. Just like any muscle, when the heart has to work hard, it gets stronger. When your heart is stronger it won't need to beat as much.

One of the benefits of regular exercise is that it will help you stay independent as you get older. By helping maintaining balance and muscle strength, you can avoid having to get around using a walker, or worse, ending up in a nursing home before your time.

Exercise can also help you maintain healthy blood sugar levels. The more you get your large muscles conditioned, the better they're going to be at taking up and metabolizing blood sugar appropriately. For this reason, your doctor may suggest you take up an exercise program if you become pre-diabetic.

Another benefit of exercise is that it can improve your mood. This won't come as a shock to those who already exercise, but for those who are not used to tying up their running shoes, they may not be aware of the endorphin rush that you get while engaging in strenuous physical activity. Exercise is a great anecdote to depression.

Does Exercise have to be intense?

The good news is that it doesn't. While you may believe that to get in shape you've got to tie up your running shoes and run as fast as you can for five miles, research has shown that in fact, you get most of the benefit in the first few minutes of exercise. So running for long periods isn't really necessary. Alternatively, exercise research has also shown that moderate exercise provides almost as many benefits. That is good enough for most of us, and you can get moderate exercise simply by walking. A rule of thumb to keep in mind is that the more moderate the exercise, the more time you should put into it. So if you're planning on a walking program, you'll probably want to walk for about 30 minutes a day 5 days a week. If you're hiking on steep mountain trails, you may need less exercise to achieve the same level of fitness. This also applies to running. Some recent research has shown that people who exercise at full blast but only do it for 1-5 minutes get the same benefit they would have gotten if they spent 20 minutes or a half hour engaged in exercise. The key isn't really to obsess over what kind of exercise "works" and what doesn't, the reality is that any kind of exercise works. So your program is to find something that you like doing and will stick to for the long term.

What Does the Science Say

When it comes to the DASH diet, the focus is on high blood pressure. So we might ask, does the DASH diet produce better results when combined with exercise? This question was asked by James Blumenthal and his colleagues in a study which compared obese subjects who followed the DASH diet and exercised with obese subjects who followed the DASH diet but who did not exercise. The subjects of the study were either pre-hypertensive or had stage 1 high blood pressure. They found that DASH diet subjects that also exercised reduced their systolic blood pressure more than 44% when compared against those who were on the DASH diet alone. Diastolic blood pressure was also better for the DASH dieters who exercised, versus those who did not, although the results were not as dramatic.

This result is so important let's state the conclusion again – People who follow the DASH diet and exercise end up with better blood pressure numbers than people who follow the DASH diet alone. This does not mean everyone on the DASH diet needs to exercise, although there are lots of reasons why everyone should exercise – but the research does confirm that exercise is at least an option that you will want to consider.

Improved Cognitive Function

One of the benefits of the DASH diet is it improves mental clarity or cognitive function. The DASH diet alone, without any exercise, can reduce the risk of developing dementia and Alzheimer's disease. The reason is that high blood pressure increases the risk of these dreaded diseases, and by reducing blood sugar the risk of getting dementia is reduced.

However, when people engage in exercise and follow the DASH diet, its been found that they have more mental focus and perform better on cognitive tests than do people who are sedentary.

Options for Exercise

There are many options available. People tend to think of exercise is jogging on a treadmill in a completely boring fashion. However, you can also consider many different activities:

- Jog outside, weather permitting.
- Take your dogs for a walk.
- Go hiking on a mountain trail.
- Go swimming.
- Take up mountain biking.
- Riding a bicycle in the city

We could list many more activities, the point is to find something that you enjoy doing. Those who exercise but do something that is not enthusiastic about doing, will get discouraged over time and end up not exercising at all.

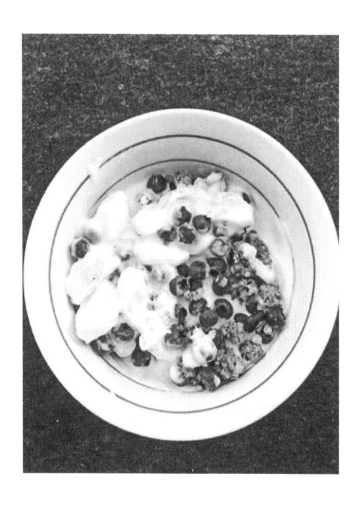

Chapter 13: 21 Day Meal Plan

The first month of a diet is normally the most challenging for people. During the initial phase of the diet, it's not entirely clear what to eat. To help get you through the first month of your diet, we've put together a simple 21-day meal plan, with suggestions for breakfast lunch and dinner.

Day 1
Breakfast

Bran flakes cereal; ¾ cup

Banana, medium sized

Milk, low-fat; 1 cup

Whole wheat bread: 1 slice

Margarine; 1tsp

Orange juice; 1 cup

Lunch

Hummus sandwich:

1 whole wheat pita bread or 2 slices of whole grain bread

½ mashed avocado

A ½ cup of arugula

3 tbsp of hummus

¼ sliced red bell pepper

¼ cup shredded carrot

¼ cup sliced cucumber

Dinner

Whole-wheat spaghetti, 1 cup; cooked

Marinara sauce, no added salt; 1 cup

Spinach for salad; 2 cups

Ranch dressing, low-fat; 1 tbsp

Whole-wheat roll, 1 small sized

Olive oil, 1 tsp

1 peach

Sparkling water (or glass of red wine for the adventurous)

Day 2

Breakfast

1 cup of steel cut oats

A ½ cup of low-fat milk

A ½ cup of low-fat cottage cheese

1 cup of applesauce

Lunch

Ham sandwich:

Honey ham, 3oz

Whole wheat bread, 2 slices

Romaine lettuce, 1 leaf, larch

Tomato, 2 slices

Mayonnaise, low-fat, 2 tsp

1 slice of low-fat provolone cheese

Broccoli, 1 cup, steamed

Orange, medium

Dinner

Trout, baked 3 oz

Broccoli, steamed, 1 cup

Whole wheat pasta, 1 cup tossed with 2 tsp. olive oil

A pinch of salt and pepper to season the pasta

1 orange

Day 3

Breakfast

1 cup of your favorite whole grain cereal, no sugar added

1 cup of milk

1 medium banana

Lunch

Tuna salad:

A ½ cup of tuna

1 leaf romaine lettuce, large

2 slices tomato

2 slices whole wheat bread

1 Tbsp low-fat mayo

1 orange

1 cup of steamed broccoli

Dinner

BBQ chicken breast:

1 baked chicken breast, with barbecue sauce

1 sweet potato

1 tsp of margarine

Salt and pepper to taste

1 cup arugula

2 tsp low-fat dressing

4 sliced cherry tomatoes

1 medium banana

Day 4

Breakfast

Orange juice, 1 cup

Fried egg

A ½ cup of fat-free, no sugar added fruit yogurt

1 cup of hot wheat cereal

Lunch

Tuna sandwich:

Tuna, 1 can

Whole wheat bread, 2 slices

Romaine lettuce, large leaf

Tomato, 2 slices

Chopped onions and celery

Mayonnaise, low-fat; 1 Tbsp

1 medium apple

Dinner

2 baked skinless chicken thighs:

Pinch of salt and pepper

Covered in shredded parmesan cheese

1 cup of stir-fried spinach

4 sliced cherry tomatoes, stir-fried with spinach

A ¼ cup of blueberries

1 cup of whole grain pasta

2 Tbsp of marinara sauce

Day 5
Breakfast

Toasted Whole wheat bread; 1 slice

Margarine; 1 tsp

Orange juice; 1 cup

Banana; medium sized

1 cup of cooked oatmeal topped with 1 tsp cinnamon and 1 tsp honey

Lunch

Lean roast beef sandwich:

3 oz roast beef

2 slices whole wheat bread

1 large leaf romaine lettuce

2 slices tomato

2 tsp mayonnaise, low-fat

1 Tbsp honey mustard

1 cup stir-fried kale and tomatoes,

1 medium orange or apple

Dinner

Beef and veggies kabob:

3 oz of lean sirloin

1 cup of cherry tomatoes, red onions, mushrooms, and sliced bell pepper

Wild rice; 1 cup

1/3 cup pecans

A ¼ cup of cranberries

1 orange

Day 6

Breakfast

1 cup of all bran or equivalent cold cereal

1 cup of milk

1 egg

1 cup of orange juice

Lunch

Tuna salad:

1 can drained tuna

2 Tbsp light mayo

¼ cup diced celery

¼ cup diced green onions

1 slice whole wheat bread

Serve tuna, celery, and green onions on top of

2 cups kale

Dinner

1 ahi tuna steak, grilled to perfection

2 cups of arugula

2 Tbsp olive oil

1 tsp lemon juice

1 medium banana

Day 7

Breakfast

2/3 cup low-fat Greek yogurt

2 tsp chia seeds

1 tsp honey

A ¼ cup of blueberries

Top yogurt with ingredients.

Lunch

Kidney bean spinach salad:

½ cup kidney beans

2 cups spinach

4 sliced grape tomatoes

A ¼ cup of diced green onions and radishes

A ¼ cup of chopped mango

2 Tbsp of red wine vinaigrette

Dinner

Garbanzo Salad:

½ diced avocado

A ½ cup of drained garbanzo beans

1 cup of diced cucumber, cherry tomatoes, and green onions

1 Tbsp sunflower seeds

2 Tbsp of low-fat salad dressing

Day 8

Breakfast

Low-fat cottage cheese; ½ cup

1 container apple sauce

1 cooked egg

1 cup of orange juice

1 banana

Lunch

Turkey breast sandwich:

Turkey (breast); 3 oz

Whole wheat bread; 2 slices

Romaine lettuce; 1 large leaf

Tomato; 2 slices

1 slice red onion

Low-Fat Mayonnaise; 2 tsp

1 slice Swiss cheese

Cauliflower, steamed; 1 cup

Banana; medium

Dinner

Baked or broiled salmon, seasoned to taste; 3 oz

1 cup arugula

1 sliced Komoto tomato

½ chopped avocado

2 Tbsp balsamic vinegar salad dressing

1 cup of cooked whole grain penne pasta, tossed in margarine and black pepper

Day 9

Breakfast

1 whole wheat bagel

1 cup of orange juice

1 fried egg

Lunch

Chicken sandwich:

Chicken breast, sliced; 3 oz

Whole wheat bread; 2 slices

Romaine lettuce; 1 large leaf

Tomato; 2 slices

Mayonnaise, low-fat; 2 tsp

Dijon mustard; 1 Tbsp

1 medium apple

Dinner

Herb-crusted baked sole

A ½ cup of wild rice

A ½ cup of steamed green beans

Whole wheat toast, 1 slice with 1 tsp. margarine

Blueberries, with chopped mint; 1 cup

1 banana

Day 10

Breakfast

Whole grain cereal; 1 cup

Low-fat cottage cheese; ½ cup

1 cup milk

Lunch

1 cup of yogurt

Quick black bean salad:

   ½ cup black beans

   ½ cup diced tomatoes

   1 cup arugula or spinach

   ¼ cup diced green onion

   ¼ cup blueberries

   2 Tbsp. low-fat Italian dressing

Dinner

Chicken and Spanish rice

1 cup cubed mango

1 cup of green peas

½ cup lettuce topped with diced tomato

Day 11

Breakfast

1 medium peach

1 cup yogurt

A ½ cup of grapefruit juice

1 slice whole wheat toast

1 tsp of margarine

Lunch

1 cup of green peas

1 cup of diced ham, mixed with 1 cup of mac and cheese (whole grain macaroni)

1 medium banana

Dinner

3 oz tilapia filet

1 tsp lemon juice

A ½ cup of brown rice

1 cup of kale sautéed with 1 Tbsp olive oil

1 Tbsp sliced almonds

1 small whole wheat roll

<u>Day 12</u>

Breakfast

1 cup of low-fat fruit yogurt

A ½ cup of orange juice

1 egg

Lunch

1 whole grain sandwich thin

A ¼ pound of lean ground turkey burger

1 slice tomato

1 slice red onion

1 slice low-fat provolone cheese

Mustard and ketchup to taste

1 medium banana

Dinner

1 chicken breast, chopped and stir-fried in 1
Tbsp olive oil

salt and pepper to taste

1 diced avocado, topped with 2 tsp of salsa

1 cup of cooked whole grain penne pasta

2 carrot sticks

Day 13
Breakfast

Low-fat milk, 1 cup

Bran flakes, 1 cup

1 slice whole wheat bread

1 tsp of margarine

1 cup of orange juice

Lunch

Turkey breast sandwich:

3 oz turkey breast

2 slices whole wheat bread

3 rings from sliced red onion

2 slices tomato

2 tsp low-fat mayo

1 slice of low-fat swiss cheese

1/2 cup mixed blueberries and raspberries

1 medium orange

Dinner

3 oz lean sirloin steak, broiled

1 cup green beans, steamed

1 medium baked potato

1 Tbsp low-fat sour cream

1 Tbsp chopped scallions

1 medium banana

1 cup milk

Day 14

Breakfast

1 slice whole wheat toast

1 tsp margarine

1 cup of low-fat cottage cheese

1 cup milk

Lunch

A ½ cup of chopped, cooked chicken

1 cup of spinach

1/3 cup of drained mandarin oranges

A ¼ cup of chopped green onion

2 Tbsp balsamic vinegar salad dressing

A ¼ cup of grated parmesan cheese

Dinner

1 can of kidney beans

1 cup of sherry wine

1 cup wild rice

1 cup of chopped white onion

2 cups of low sodium chicken broth

1 cup of chopped celery

A ¼ cup of sliced carrots

Day 15
Breakfast
¾ cup bran flakes

1 cup milk

1 whole wheat bagel

Lunch
Mixed meat sandwich:

1 oz each of turkey breast, ham, and roast beef

2 slices whole wheat bread

1 large leaf romaine lettuce

2 slices tomato

1 slice provolone cheese

2 tsp mayonnaise, low-fat

1 Tbsp Dijon mustard

1 cup sautéed spinach,

1 medium orange

Dinner

1/2 can garbanzo beans, cooked with ½ cup
diced tomatoes, 1 minced garlic, 2 Tbsp chopped
basil leaves, 1 tsp. lemon juice in a saucepan

1 cup cooked whole grain orzo

Day 16
Breakfast

Steel cut oats, ½ cup

Whole wheat bagel; 1 whole

Margarine; 1 tsp

Orange

1 cup milk

Lunch

Whole wheat bread, 2 slices

Cheddar cheese, 1 slice

3 oz sliced chicken breast

1 large leaf romaine lettuce

1 Tbsp low-fat mayo

3 rings of sliced red onion

Tomato; 2 slices

1 cup of orange juice

Banana; medium sized

Dinner

1 cup of whole wheat spaghetti

A ½ cup of chopped shrimp

1 Tbsp capers

6 sliced cherry tomatoes

3 Tbsp parmesan cheese

½ cup marinara sauce

1 cup spinach/kale mix, sautéed

1 Tbsp sliced almonds

Day 17

Breakfast

1 cup yogurt

1 cup mixed fruit

1 egg

Lunch

Spinach salad with garbanzo beans:

1 cup spinach

½ cup garbanzo beans

¼ cup sliced mushrooms

A ¼ cup of grated carrots

4 sliced cherry tomatoes

1 Tbsp sliced almonds

½ cup mandarin oranges

1 Tbsp low-fat salad dressing

Dinner

3 oz broiled chicken breast, topped with 1 Tbsp
spicy barbecue sauce

1 cup steamed green beans

1 medium sweet potato

1 tsp margarine

Salt and pepper to taste

1 medium orange

Day 18
Breakfast

1 pear, sliced, topped with ground cinnamon

1 slice whole wheat toast

1 tsp margarine

1 cup milk

Lunch
1 cup Greek yogurt

1 can salmon, drained and flaked

1 whole wheat pita bread

2 tsp dill

½ cup watercress

1 tsp lemon juice

Dinner
Grilled flank steak, marinated in low sodium
teriyaki sauce

1 cup steamed green beans

1 cup of whole grain pasta, tossed in olive oil and
black pepper

1 cup milk

1 medium banana

Day 19
Breakfast
1 cup of mixed fruit

1 cup of yogurt

1 bran muffin

1 tsp margarine

Lunch

Ham and cheddar sandwich:

3 oz black forest ham

Whole wheat bread, 2 slices

1 large leaf romaine lettuce

Mayonnaise, low-fat, 2 tsp

1 slice cheddar cheese

1 cup steamed broccoli

1 cup of green grapes

Dinner

1 cup cooked quinoa

½ cup diced cucumber

¼ cup pitted black olives

¼ cup chopped red onion

¼ cup crumbled feta cheese

2 tbsp chopped parsley

2 Tbsp olive oil

Pinch of salt, black pepper to taste

Cooked and sliced skinless chicken breast

Day 20

Breakfast

½ cup blueberries

1 slice whole wheat toast

1 tsp. margarine

1 cup milk

1 cup yogurt

Lunch

3oz cup chopped, cooked chicken

1 whole wheat tortilla

2 Tbsp mayo

½ tsp curry powder

1 Tbsp salsa

½ avocado, chopped

Dinner

3 oz sirloin steak

1 cup spinach

2 sliced grape tomatoes

¼ cup grated parmesan cheese

¼ cup chopped red onion

1 baked potato

1 tsp margarine

1 Tbsp low-fat sour cream

Day 21

Breakfast

Instant oatmeal, ½ cup

Wheat Bagel; whole

Peanut butter, 1 Tbsp

Banana, 1 medium

Milk, 1 cup

Lunch

Turkey breast sandwich:

  Turkey breast, 3 oz

Whole wheat bread, 2 slices

Romaine lettuce, 1 large leaf

Tomato, 2 slices

Mayonnaise, low-fat, 1 tsp

Dijon mustard, 1 Tbsp

Broccoli, steamed, 1 cup

Orange, 1 medium sized

Dinner

Baked cod, 3 oz

Wild rice, 1 cup

A ½ cup of cooked spinach

2 tsp canola oil

1 Tbsp slivered almonds

1 small whole wheat roll

1 small cookie

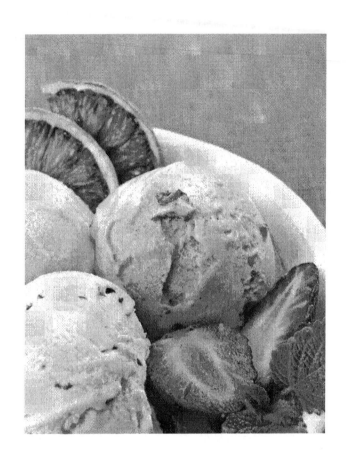

Conclusion

Thank you for taking the time to read this book on the DASH diet! We sincerely hope that the book was educational and helpful.

We also hope that you will take the lessons of the DASH diet to heart. Namely that you can take charge of your own health. Remember what grandma said – you are what you eat.

And it's true!

Medical professionals are finally starting to realize that diet is more important than ever imagined. The diet you eat has a strong influence on nearly all aspects of your health, but it's most influential on your future risks of heart disease and diabetes. Moreover, with the research that led to the development of the DASH diet, it was found that the nutrients we eat can even determine whether or not we have high blood pressure.

If you have high blood pressure, be sure to speak with your doctor before making radical changes in your diet, and take up this diet only under a doctors supervision. It's so effective that your continued use of medication will have to be carefully monitored.

If you found this book useful and informative, please drop by and give us a review!

Thanks for reading, and good luck with your health!

71119517R00120

Made in the USA
Columbia, SC
24 August 2019